parenting forever

Elizabeth Green, MBBS (Hons), FRACP, is a paediatrician and parent. She graduated from Melbourne University in 1982 and has a vast and diverse bank of clinical experience. This incorporates city and rural general practice and being a flying doctor in Kalgoorlie, Western Australia. Working with children in remote parts of Australia sparked her passion for paediatrics. She qualified as a paediatrician in 1997 and now works in private paediatric practice in Perth.

Dr Green is a member of the Neurodevelopmental and Behavioural Paediatric Society of Australasia (NBPSA) and advocates for childhood. She has a recognised and respected media voice on topical issues that impact on kids and families. These include social and technological change, anxiety, autism, ADHD, performance and learning pressures, and rising mental health issues.

parenting is forever

a paediatrician's
tips for parents,
teachers
and carers

dr elizabeth green

UWA PUBLISHING

First published in 2017 by
UWA Publishing
Crawley, Western Australia 6009
www.uwap.uwa.edu.au

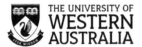

THE UNIVERSITY OF
WESTERN
AUSTRALIA

National Library of Australia Cataloguing-in-Publication entry
Green, Elizabeth, author.
Parenting is forever: a paediatrician's tips for parents,
teachers and carers / Elizabeth Green.
ISBN: 9781742589565 (paperback)
Parenting—--Handbooks, manuals, etc.
Child rearing—Handbooks, manuals, etc.
Parent and child.
Child psychology—Handbooks, manuals, etc.

Cover design by Upside Creative
Typeset in Bembo by Lasertype
Printed by Lightning Source

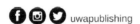 uwapublishing

This book is dedicated to
my family and yours
and to the third carrot on the left.

FOREWORD

One of the roles and privileges of a developmental paediatrician is to be an advocate for the developmental wellbeing of children and young people.

Dr Green is strongly committed to such advocacy, based on her own experiences of parenting and her professional knowledge and observations in an increasingly complex society. Modern life, with its challenges and anxiety, has potential to interfere with developmental progress.

There is a concerning rise in developmental difficulties. Obesity has increased. Learning problems carry the associated stress and anxiety of school failure. There is an increase in attention deficit disorders and autism. In this book, Dr Green explains and gives practical advice on these developmental concerns.

Scientific research acknowledges the importance of the first 3 to 5 years of life for the neurological secure attachment between child and caregiver. There is a partnership between 'nature and nurture'. Secure attachment has a positive preventive influence on developmental outcome. Conversely, difficulties with attachment and adverse events are found to be causally related to health concerns in adult life.

Further, we now know the neurological influences in the early years. Dr Jack Shonkoff wrote, in 2006:

> 100 billion nerve cells are present at birth – most of these are unconnected. Each neuron may eventually connect to as many as 15,000

other neurones. By the age of three, a child's brain has 1,000 trillion connections. By late adolescence one-third of these synapses have been discarded. Forming and reinforcing these connections are the key tasks of early brain development.

Early brain growth and maturation is a complex neurological event. I muse on how, with such dynamic activity, the majority of young children are within the normal developmental range. Shonkoff continues:

> The early years of life matter because the ongoing interaction between early experiences and gene expression affects the architecture of the maturing brain. As it emerges, the quality of that architecture establishes either a sturdy or a fragile foundation for all the learning, health and behaviour that follows. Nurturing and responsive relationships build healthy brain architecture that provides a strong foundation for learning, behaviour and health. When protective relationships are not provided, elevated levels of stress hormones disrupt brain architecture by impairing cell growth and interfering with the formation of healthy neural circuits.

We now have sound scientific knowledge to encourage the capacity of attachment to enhance developmental outcomes. One relevant program to assist parents and carers in secure attachment in the early years is the 'Circle of Security'. This is an established and international parenting intervention. It teaches parents and carers how to better recognise, listen and respond to the needs of the child. A child's attachment to their primary carer is affirmed and their emotional security and behaviour improves.

While meaning well, some concerns raised by parents, teachers and carers can increase anxiety for adults and children. The world has become more stressful for young families. This stress can be one of the factors that makes it difficult for children to feel secure, though otherwise healthy and following a normal pathway.

The African quote, 'It takes a whole village to raise a child' is well known. However, I would ask, 'What kind of village these days?'

The village I hope to see encourages healthy feeding, restful sleep, age-appropriate exercise, play-based learning, early literacy and language exposure, lullabies and secure attachment – all coupled with community support and accessible services. Prevention should be foremost in our thinking. This facilitates the early identification and assessment of developmental concerns and leads to age-appropriate intervention. Not only are these approaches right for parents and their children, but in the 'village' there is a need for support and information for allied health and educators.

Current health and developmental concerns for children are obesity, clinical anxiety, learning disorders, ADHD and autism. Dr Green describes these topical issues clearly. She gives practical advice on strategies and approaches to help manage and understand the stress and difficulty in having a child who doesn't follow a 'normal' developmental trajectory.

With honest sharing and passion, Dr Green imparts her knowledge, wisdom and understanding of social change as it relates to the interests of raising children through to adulthood. She informs, reassures and encourages the confident engagement in what is a 'forever' privilege and demand.

Clinical Professor Trevor Parry, AMCitWA

Dr Trevor Parry was made a Member of the Order of Australia in 2012 for his lifetime of service given to improve the health and wellbeing of Western Australian children.

CONTENTS

INTRODUCTION

Parenting is not a competition. It is not about who finds it harder – parents or grandparents. Being a mother or father, aunt, uncle or grandparent is a role of privilege. You will not perform it perfectly. There will be times when you make poor choices. But, if you learn from mistakes, you become a better parent.

Children also learn through failure. They develop emotional resilience, cope with disappointment and find the determination to 'have a go'. Then, they succeed.

This book is about how to stand alongside your child. To help them when they stumble and fall. Parenting is for the long term. Your trek starts when you prepare for parenthood. It continues even after your child emerges as a young adult. Parents want their children to be happy, emotionally secure, socially competent and employable.

Children now live in a busy, anxious digital world. This has created complexity and new challenges for parents. It has always been hard to raise children. Any grandparent or mentor will attest to that. Raising two daughters is the most difficult thing I do. Being a paediatrician who cares for kids who struggle to walk, talk, play and learn is easy!

My first tip is to accept regret, adapt to change and enjoy your children. Live life in the moment. Look back through the rear-vision mirror and you will miss your child's dreams.

Make time to enjoy your baby, toddler, child, adolescent or young adult. Don't be afraid of parenthood. You will be the same person after having a child, but with a broader life perspective. Knowledge is empowering. It enables you to parent with confidence. There are no prescriptive rules on how to parent. The parent–child relationship is yours. It is unique.

This book describes common medical and mental health problems that afflict children and families. Anxiety, attention deficit hyperactivity disorder (ADHD), specific learning disorders (SLDs), autism and eating disorders are conditions worth knowing about. There is a reasonable chance your child will meet one of these 'cruel friends'.

You may have had school learning difficulties, concentration and listening problems or have been an anxious child. Did parental anxiety, anger, depression, separation, alcohol and drug abuse or domestic violence impact on your childhood? If you tick any of these 'risk' factors, ensure that your own mental health is robust when you have a child.

Consider what 'normal' child development means. Look at pivotal childhood stages through childhood 'SPECS', an acronym for *S*peech, language and communication; *P*hysical fitness, fine and gross motor coordination; *E*motional resilience; *C*ognitive growth; and *S*ocial competency. These areas define childhood milestones. They determine when your child smiles, talks and walks. It is when they read, write, ask questions and play.

Most children and teenagers experience anxiety. Some parents still carry the mental distress of this condition from shattered childhoods. Anxiety is a 'cruel' friend for kids and families. It takes the fun out of childhood. Read about this disorder. Confront anxiety and you can cope with it. Ignore stress in the early childhood years and it will rebound in adolescence.

I share my expertise about children and their physical, social, emotional and academic development. Not to overwhelm parents, teachers and those who value children, but to empower them with knowledge. Relax. You may feel as if your world is falling apart when you are told, 'Your child has autism or ADHD'. But, it won't. You never have to parent alone!

Don't be afraid of the 3-year-old who performs their act of angry, sad and mad in front of you. Let your teenager 'vent' by screaming at you. Avoid a reactive, impulsive conversation. Any communication beats the silence of the depressed adolescent.

Try parenting – if this is your choice. Parent together or with a support person. Otherwise everything falls apart. Help others if you don't choose to parent. Be the best aunt, brother or cousin.

Respect and believe in your child. Value them and be kind. Remember this, and you will give your child a good start in life. Good luck!

Part 1

Pondering parenthood

'I can't do it alone,'
Said the Cat in the Hat.
'It is good I have some one
To help me,' he said.
'Right here in my hat
On the top of my head!'

The Cat in the Hat Comes Back – Dr Seuss

Parenting choices

Have children, don't have children, but whichever choice you make, stick to it and enjoy life.

If you have ever owned a cat and found this challenging, don't rush into parenting. Raising a child is even harder and it's for the long term.

I was never a cat lover. I am allergic to cats. They make my skin itch and turn into a collage of red lumps and bumps. I sneeze, wheeze, and stare at them through angry, puffed-up eyes. They look at me with disdain and with a dismissive wave of their tails, they are gone.

One day I arrived home to find two fluffy balls of feline mischief hiding behind our washing machine. My husband had succumbed to the persistent pleas of our daughters to rescue two ordinary kittens from a cat shelter. He failed the first lesson of parenting. Be a rock. But, I have learned that parenting benefits from flexibility when practised in a calm, consistent and reflective way.

The rules for having a well-behaved cat are the same as for growing emotionally secure and resilient children. You start with a raw bundle of life made up of great genetic diversity. You place this in an unfamiliar environment and wait for the adult to emerge. This requires great patience. As a parent to your pet or child you can influence how this process will evolve. The love and nurture you provide in the very early months and years affect the outcome.

I have learned to be a great cat parent of two extraordinary cats. They have taught me nearly as much about parenting as my own children. As a bonus, my cat allergy has pretty much resolved. I am not a perfect parent, but every day I try to be a better one. I am prepared to listen and learn, to fail, and through failure succeed.

Parental challenges

I wish someone had given me a book on how to meet the challenges of parenthood.

Chance and circumstance can dictate parenting. Genetics, environment, life events, our own childhood experiences and those of our parents influence the way we raise children. Success is a subjective judgement.

Parenting is about looking forward, trying harder and letting go of what has passed. It is about the impact of society's culture on the child and the child's perception of being in the family they are given; not always the family they choose.

Functional families don't always understand the distress of those families who struggle because of mental distress, difficult family dynamics or severe financial hardship. The most competent families can find themselves in chaos when unexpected events change their life trajectory. There are no perfect or normal families. The best families are kind, empathic and have healthy genes.

The recipe for raising children has become complex. Children and parents haven't changed. But the world we live in has. Homes and communities are anxious places. Parents are overwhelmed with responsibility. They feel judged and disempowered.

Most parents want to bumble along, live a less pressured lifestyle, learn as they go and raise happy children. Simple is best.

We outsource parenting from the time our children are born. This has made parents feel insecure and inadequate. If parents are empowered they parent better.

Insular family units, designer children, pampered pets and indulgent parenting transform the normality of life. Overpraise and control of children smothers their resilience and sets them up for failure. Posting seconds of fame online is the ultimate adolescent dream. Narcissistic goals have drowned reality. Digital playgrounds and workplaces are the result of the social shift we have all helped create.

Social shift is the result of evolved technologies and frenetic lifestyles. It changes the way we talk, listen and socially connect with each other. This 'shift' replaces kindness with selfishness, hypersexualises our children and takes respect out of relationships. Children sense and feel these emotions and become anxious.

When we need to ask, 'How do I play with my child?', it is time to vary the direction of our social compass. Our priority is to restore common sense, consistent rules, stillness, love, compassion, imagination and play to childhood. Instead, we seek a prescriptive solution on how to parent.

I have been the mother of two daughters for twenty years, and a paediatrician for longer. I look after children with neurodevelopmental and behavioural disorders. This means I care for kids with problems talking, walking, learning, socialising, playing and being happy.

My work helps me understand the pivotal steps in a child's emotional, social and cognitive development as they grow towards adolescence and adult life. To see how the imperfections of the child and their families can become their strengths. Look beyond flaws and see what our children can do, rather than what they can't.

Malcolm Fraser famously paraphrased the quote from George Bernard Shaw: 'Life is not meant to be easy, my child; but take courage: it can be delightful'. An imperfect or difficult life can be much more interesting.

Life progresses through a number of sliding doors. They lead us forward. Life can't be lived in reverse.

You don't parent alone. Your network is 'the village'. It assists you to build the safety nets that catch your children and throw them back into the world. It helps you raise children with strong emotional and social resilience.

Children need strategies in their toolkit to build social and emotional competency. This helps them achieve to their optimal ability. Failure to instil these values during the early childhood years makes a child vulnerable to mental distress in later childhood or adult life. This includes anxiety and depression, eating disorders, obsessive-compulsive disorder, self-harm behaviours and sibling rivalry. Some families have genes which make them more likely to have significant mental health disorders. These are bipolar and major depression, borderline personality, generalised anxiety and schizophrenia.

Children who are victims of domestic violence, including overt and covert physical, sexual and emotional abuse, are at risk of developmental trauma. A child's emotional resilience is the protective body armour they put on during the early years. They will need this. You want it to be strong.

Adults have a duty of care to uphold the rights of the child within homes, schools and places where children are sent without their consent. These include hospitals, boarding schools, foster homes and refugee camps. We must listen more carefully to the voices of these vulnerable children.

Parenting is no longer a gender or biologically determined role. It is a shared responsibility that requires us to focus on the child, hear their needs and work out who can best meet them.

Don't be afraid of children. They are fun, engaging, insightful and challenging. Parenting children is never boring. Let's share this story together.

Parental perspective

Remember to breathe when caught up in the whirlwind that can engulf childhood. It is important that in an era painted with doom and gloom we do not catastrophise life. If parents fall into this trap, their children will sensationalise and fear life. There are too many negative families who worry about life scenarios that do not eventuate.

Paediatricians and parents have the positive role of building childhood resilience. This will help children and adolescents approach life with purpose and hope. 'And will you succeed?' Dr Seuss says. 'Yes! You will, indeed! (98 and ¾ per cent guaranteed.)'

Social shift

If you are the parent, grandparent, mentor or educator of Generation Z you need to consider the social and technological change that defines this cohort. 'Gen Z' are kids now, born in the 2000s.

Bringing up children today differs significantly from previous generations because of the development and expansion of the internet since the early 1990s. This technological revolution led to the emergence of an electronic surge of information, social prying, unrealistic expectations and anxiety.

Our social shift has disrupted family cohesion by interrupting 'face-to-face' conversation. Social media is the preferred mode of communication for children and adolescents. Parents who don't keep up with technology are socially excluded from their kids.

Social discourse is punctuated by 'digital darts', bits of digital information fired at us, followed by texts, 'selfies' and the electronic pings and pongs from email inboxes. These electronic distractions have made parents ineffective and families time-poor.

Parents need to take charge and restore life's balance. They can do this by instructing children how to use technology safely and responsibly to learn, create and innovate.

Social shift has been stealthily creeping upon us over the last ten to fifteen years. It has displaced common sense and resulted in an unhealthy balance in child rearing. Electronic and social media, school commitments and the external pressure of extracurricular activities control families.

This disruption to our social ebb and flow has become trans-generational. How can parents who have not been taught social rules impart life skills to their own children? If parents do not have self-respect and self-discipline, then neither will their children. These values are best learned within the home and when children are very young.

In Melbourne recently I caught the train to visit family. A young mother, accompanied by her friend, stepped into my carriage. She was struggling with her shopping bags and small child who was lying back in his stroller. As we approached the train station, the young child yelled out 'Chips'. The mother ignored him until he screamed, 'Give me the fucking chips'. The mother laughed at the comment made by her child and repeated it. 'Did you hear that? He said "Give me the fucking chips"'. I felt sadness for that child's loss of opportunity.

Social shift has created sad, mad (emotionally dysregulated), bad (oppositional), angry and anxious children. It has resulted in reactive, angry, controlling and over-protective parenting. Parents don't let their kids learn through failure. They 'rescue' and 'smother' them. This stops kids taking risks – from having a go at life.

To raise children to be happy, emotionally resilient adults, able to form stable relationships and embrace life, parenting has to change. A child responds to positive parenting and acknowledgement for trying. Combative, angry and impulsive parenting causes oppositional behaviours. Discipline is best when delivered in a calm, consistent, fair and reflective way.

Parents benefit from 'pause and think time'. This helps them make rational decisions and good choices. Good parenting won't work in the middle of a child's meltdown. A child has to first settle down. This is when parenting skills can work.

Part 2

The years 'BC' – life before children

I love you right up to the moon – AND BACK.

Big Nutbrown Hare, *Guess How Much I Love You*

Written by Sam McBratney, illustrated by Anita Jeram

Thinking babies?

Parenthood means babies

Sometimes we stumble into parenthood hoping that the romance and emotion of having a baby is enough preparation. Our lives are too busy to talk about the responsibilities and duties of care linked with parenthood. Planning a family should be part of the discussion before committing your heart and soul to another person.

We spend more time researching where we want to live, the type of home we will purchase and how we are going to keep our own careers viable whilst juggling the responsibilities of parenthood. Babies can be the afterthought.

Some professional couples put off having a baby. A child means uncertainty. They don't like the thought of losing control, or the routine in their lives. They worry about having an 'abnormal' child.

The decision to have a baby requires you to rethink career goals and life expectations. Throw perfect and anxious out the window before you have children.

Prepare and plan for parenthood. This is a lifetime commitment.

Salty cakes – practice doesn't bake perfect

Raising a child is like baking a cake. Cakes are not perfect but they can be great. Childhood is the same.

Making cakes and having children requires thought, planning, preparation and perseverance. Most importantly, it demands time. There is a sense of pride when the cake we make, bake and ice is chosen and devoured. No one complains about the lopsided cake that tastes good. So, why are we so prescriptive and critical when it comes to children?

Our narcissistic society promotes power. This has contributed to our gender gap which makes it hard for women who are sole parents to raise children. We have shifted expectations about bringing up children to heady levels. By lifting the bar on what to expect from parenthood we have created a generation of anxious and insecure parents. We have set ourselves up for failure. No wonder there are people who are reluctant or choose not to raise children. 'Get out as early as you can, and don't have any kids yourself', says Philip Larkin in his oft-quoted poem, 'This Be The Verse'.

You don't have to have children

Some people can't, or don't want to, have children. But most people have children or will trip over them in their lives. It helps to try to understand them. They might even get to like them.

Each of us holds the power to make a difference to a child. This is a great responsibility and one we must honour.

Some iconic figures have chosen not to have children. The late Colleen McCullough, author of *The Thorn Birds*, said a definite 'no' to children. Andrew Denton interviewed her on his TV program, *Enough Rope,* in September 2007. When asked about why she chose not to have children, her reply was, 'I don't much like children'. She also alluded to her own 'ghastly' childhood.

A medical colleague of mine is a highly qualified and clinically discerning medical practitioner. Her life path has not included children. She has been a mentor to many children and their families.

Whilst my friend embraced a life without the challenges of childhood, another peer found it difficult. Although trying for children she had not been able to conceive. She expressed her disappointment to me one day by saying, 'Not having children is like not being invited to a birthday party'. If she had attended some of the children's birthday parties that I have been to, she might be glad not to have received an invitation. Sometimes there are no words to shift sadness. It is best to listen silently.

Nature and nurture

They fuck you up, your mum and dad.
They may not mean to, but they do.
They fill you with the faults they had
And add some extra, just for you.

'This Be The Verse' – Philip Larkin

Epigenetics

Epigenetics is a complex and evolving science about how our genes are more than just DNA, the genetic material that programs what we look like. We are learning that external biochemical, environmental or biophysical factors can change the way that genes work by making them switch their function on or off. The ability for genes to be modified so that they express different physical characteristics despite having the same DNA occurs in all of our cells. It is genetically inherited across generations.

Scientists are now doing studies on how external factors, such as maternal stress, nutrition, infection and tobacco smoking around the time of conception, affect the foetus (unborn baby). It is too early to know whether this knowledge could be used in future insurance or legal claims. That remains an ethical question.

Epigenetics explains why identical twins with the same DNA can have a different expression of mental or physical disease when subject to varying environments. One twin, for example, may develop type 1 diabetes during childhood whilst the other doesn't.

You can think about epigenetics as two cakes baked with the same mixture. One cake is lightly browned and well baked when you remove it from the oven. The other will be undercooked if it has been baked at a lower temperature, even in the same oven. They are the same cakes but have different outcomes, depending on the conditions of their environment.

Experts in the evolving science of epigenetics report that both overweight and underweight babies have a higher risk of developing diabetes in later life. These observations make us look more closely at the potential for the early intrauterine environment of the baby to have a long-term impact on its future health.

We know that maternal mental and physical health affects our child. We can take charge of our adult life. Plan and nurture. Raise healthy children.

Mothers who have a child with a disability or a later mental health problem always express their feelings of guilt pertaining to their pregnancy experience. They regret the busyness and stress of this time. They reveal that they didn't want to have a child with a disability, had fertility problems or didn't expect to fall pregnant.

Mothers recall with clarity, tears and emotion seeing their child with an obvious chromosomal abnormality such as Down syndrome or cleft lip and palate. They blame themselves for consuming alcohol when pregnant or for getting the flu in early pregnancy. These are things past. If you are a guilt-ridden mother, tilt your rear-vision mirror away and look forwards through the front window. That is where your life is heading now.

The new science of epigenetics is very exciting and we will hear lots more about it. Epigenetics introduces new science to the old 'nature versus nurture' discussion. It considers the significance of external environmental factors affecting the developing neural wiring of the embryo, infant and child during the critical years of early child development. Mothers should keep this science in perspective. It is not meant to frighten you. It is there to help you prepare as best you can for your baby. That is all you can do.

Sometimes, despite the best pregnancy preparation, a child is born with an unexpected chromosomal or genetic disorder which we can't fix. This is when we need strong emotional resilience and the support of partners, family and other village members.

The bun in the oven

Babies are like buns in the oven. Their external environment affects them. If the oven is too hot the buns burn. If your baby has a sub-optimal uterine environment, they may be born too small or too big. You can't always prevent this as a mother, even with the best antenatal care. If babies are tightly packaged in the uterus and don't have enough wriggle room they may be born with positional neck problems such as torticollis (wryneck), or feet and hip problems. We don't cook perfect buns or cakes and we can't make perfect babies. We all have genetic flaws programmed into our DNA. This keeps us unique and allows us to evolve.

One of the problems with having access to knowledge and technology is that we can overprepare and overthink our baby's progress during pregnancy. We can become so focused on our unborn child that we neglect to care for maternal needs and those of a partner or other children.

I am often asked why we are seeing so much anxiety in our daily lives. Anxiety starts from the womb. Women are choosing to have babies later, which places them under a biological time pressure. When women fall pregnant they are constantly worrying about their chance of miscarriage and whether their baby will be healthy.

Their fears are reinforced by the huge amount of information relating to pregnancy and parenting. Antenatal tests are available to tell women what their likelihood is of giving birth to a child with Down syndrome or with a brain, spine or heart defect.

Ultrasounds can bring great joy when they confirm a viable pregnancy and demonstrate normal serial growth of a baby. They can create stress when they show indeterminate gender, possible cleft lip or palate deformity, or developmental brain variants such as choroid plexus cysts. These are usually benign and resolve during pregnancy.

Women need to be informed about all the diagnostic screening tests available to them so that they can make an informed decision about how often they are going to open the oven door and test their 'bun in the oven'.

Obstetricians are much more focused on providing this information to families, partly because of the high medico-legal risk if they don't. There are helpful online sites that provide accurate and detailed information to parents about screening tests and procedures during pregnancy and the newborn period. I have included some of these under 'Helpful reading'.

If you are planning a pregnancy try not to be overwhelmed with the vast volume of information and data available to you. There are probably too many choices. This leads to indecision, anxiety and even guilt. Be selective with the resources you use and seek support that is most appropriate for your situation.

Trust your obstetrician and midwife and do some selective research on the internet. Remember to enjoy the experience of being pregnant. Look forward to being a parent. You have been given an amazing privilege and opportunity.

Baby talk

Communication is important – talk with your partner

Planning a pregnancy means that you want a child. Your partner or support person has to want one too. A strong relationship is a good start to parenthood. If you recognise partner problems, work on these before having children. One of the first questions an obstetrician should ask is, 'How is your marriage or your partnership?' Of course they don't. It is up to you to ask yourself this question.

Having a baby won't solve relationship difficulties. It can make them worse. Talk with your partner about the expectations of parenthood. This discussion should take place before having a baby. When the baby comes first, still talk and support!

Timing is critical

One of the baby myths I hear in my work with families is that age is not considered a barrier for having children. Professional couples are surprised when informed that fertility rates drop with increased maternal age.

Having a baby at 40 years of age is harder than when you were 20 years old. However, being young doesn't guarantee a successful pregnancy. Allow enough time to plan a pregnancy. Some couples wait four or five years before a confirmed pregnancy. They require fertility assistance. Face the possibility of adoption or surrogacy options. It can be more challenging being an older parent, although many mothers manage this role beautifully.

Family ties – history is important

Couples have vastly different social and cultural backgrounds. The emotional baggage of your own childhood and transgenerational problems affect the way you parent. Family history gives clues to the genetic risks of your child. Combined with specific environmental factors, your child is at greater risk of developing mental distress if you have a history of mental health issues. Anxiety, depression, eating disorders, bipolar disorder and addiction run in families. So do autism, attention deficit hyperactivity disorder (ADHD) and specific learning disorders (SLDs) such as dyslexia, dyscalculia or dysgraphia.

Some families have a significant cardiovascular disease risk such as death from a heart attack under the age of 40 years, or high cholesterol levels. Others have autoimmune disorders such as diabetes, rheumatoid arthritis, thyroid disease and immunodeficiency disorders which make children susceptible to infection. Bleeding disorders, including haemophilia and Von Willebrand disease. Haemochromatosis, an iron storage disorder; thalassaemia, a blood disorder; and cystic fibrosis, a chronic respiratory and gut disease. It is important to know about family history.

This is imperative in families with a strong history of cancer. Some faulty genes are linked with a high lifelong chance of cancer. The BRCA gene mutation is associated with an increase in a small percentage of breast and ovarian cancers. Actor Angelina Jolie has the inherited BRCA1 mutation. She has given women greater awareness of this risk factor.

We don't often ask or consider the potential impact of family history on our own children. It is usually a topic avoided by women before committing to a relationship. Sometimes this is not a bad thing. We can ask and know too much. When we embrace life we accept a certain amount of risk, uncertainty and challenge. I hope we are never in a position where we micromanage romance and relationships.

Having a baby and testing friendships

Friendship groups change when you first embark on parenthood. They consist of those who have or are having children and those who don't. Social gatherings centre on the intricacies of breastfeeding, changing nappies and pram brands. With time, this temporary segregation sorts itself out and you mix with friends who are helpful and positive in your life and avoid those who are not, irrespective of whether your friends are child-credentialed.

If you are separated physically by state or country borders from extended family, keep connected with them. This is facilitated by technology such as Skype, which is embraced by many grandparents. Use your pregnancy time to upskill on technology or take an online course if you haven't completed tertiary qualifications. This is the best time to start. It is very hard to undertake tertiary studies, even part-time, when you have a young child.

Healthy starts

Healthy lifestyle – giving your baby the best start you can

He who is devoid of kindness is devoid of grace.

Arabian proverb

Children are raised by parents and proxy parents such as grand-parents and mentors. Professional advice from paediatricians, psychologists, psychiatrists and teachers can disempower parents. It can catastrophise parenting. Trust your parental intuition. Add it to the wealth of knowledge you can access about raising your child.

A pregnancy can be planned, overplanned or unexpected. Once you know that you are going to have a baby you have parental responsibility.

There are a few things worth considering to help you parent better:

Values – Kindness, grace, compassion, tolerance, selflessness and steadfastness are needed to raise happy and emotionally secure children.

'Mindfulness' and 'heartfulness' – Self-reflection is about understanding and caring for self. Emotionally strong parents provide good role models and instil emotional resilience in children.

Empathy – Walk in the shoes of your child. Learn to interpret and understand their behaviour rather than react to it. Do this from day one!

Common sense – You will never be a 'perfect' parent. Just be the best parent you can. Trust your intuition and common sense. This is a scarcity in hectic lives.

Practical sense – You need to do some financial planning and preparation work. Find a doctor and midwife that you respect and trust. They will care for you in your pregnancy and deliver your baby or babies.

Healthy lifestyle – This means no alcohol, no smoking, no self-medicating with abusive substances and regular exercise. Minimal stress is mandatory. You don't need to eat for two. This just piles on the kilos. One drink is not okay. Seek help if you are anxious, afraid or depressed.

Social connectivity – Now is the time to say sorry and reconnect with family.

Relationship – Talk with your partner. Listen to their view on parenting.

Consistency – Decide on how you will discipline, guide and love your child. Make sure you are 'on the same page' before you are a parent. This allows you to practise consistent, reflective and fair parenting.

What's good for your baby?

Keep parenting plans simple

A healthy life balance is good for you and for your baby. You may have to rethink 'having it all' when you choose parenthood. As a prospective parent you will be told from multiple sources what you should eat and what can't be consumed. Too many decisions create anxiety. This is what happens to many parents. They are anxious before they even have their baby!

Stick to the five healthy food groups

Dairy sources provide calcium. Fruit and vegetables contain vitamins and dietary fibre. Grains and cereals also have fibre and nutrients. Lean meats, poultry, fish, eggs, tofu, nuts and seeds have high levels of protein. Vegetables and legumes are good for vitamins such as folate.

Maintain a healthy weight range

Monitor weight gain during pregnancy. Do this by eating sensibly and exercising regularly. There is great support to help you keep these goals. Just ask.

Dietary modification

This is required for food intolerances and allergies. Vegetarian and vegan life choices pose nutritional challenges during pregnancy. Medical conditions such as diabetes and coeliac disease (wheat, oats, rye and barley intolerance) will benefit from a dietician's input.

Dietary supplements

Start these when you are planning a pregnancy. Include iron, folate (folic acid), iodine, vitamin D, probiotics and fish oil. Vitamin B_{12} levels can be low in mothers who are vegetarian or vegan. Caution and medical advice applies for iodine supplements if you have a problem with your thyroid gland. It is best to avoid fish oil if you have a severe seafood allergy or bleeding disorder.

Iron

Research informs us why dietary supplements are advisable before and during pregnancy. Many young women have low iron stores and can develop anaemia during this time. A low blood count makes them pale, tired and short of breath when they exercise.

Babies and mothers need a diet which is rich in iron so that they can make healthy blood cells, stay well and grow a healthy baby. An iron-containing diet includes meat, chicken, fish, cereals, wholegrain breads, green leafy vegetables, legumes and nuts. The richest source of iron is from red meat – not from spinach!

Folate

In 1989, Professor Fiona Stanley and Professor Carol Bower, Western Australian scientists, showed that dietary folate, a B-group vitamin found in leafy green vegetables, legumes, cereals and wholegrain breads, could significantly reduce neural tube defects, known as spina bifida. This condition is due to deformities of the lower part of the spinal cord and results in bladder, bowel and lower limb dysfunction.

This innovative research has had a positive impact on our public health. Australia now fortifies all bread (wheat flour) products with folate.

A daily folate supplement of 500 micrograms together with a daily dietary intake of 600 micrograms of folate is recommended prior to and during pregnancy. Most pharmacies can advise which folate supplement is suitable for pregnancy.

Iodine

Iodine is an essential trace element found in saltwater fish, shellfish, seaweed, dairy, eggs, soy milk, soy sauce and iodised table salt. Natural sea salt contains only small amounts of iodine.

The body does not make iodine, but needs it for the production of thyroid hormone. This is important for normal brain, heart, muscle and metabolic function. When your body makes insufficient thyroid hormone, your thyroid gland, at the front of your neck, enlarges into a goitre and becomes underactive (hypothyroid). This makes you feel tired, cold and lethargic, and may result in a slow pulse, dry hair, constipation and fuzzy thinking.

In the pregnant or nursing mother, iodine deficiency has been associated with miscarriage, stillbirth, preterm delivery and congenital abnormalities. In severe cases, a baby can have intellectual disability, deafness, altered muscle tone and short stature.

Women planning a pregnancy or women who are pregnant or lactating should take an iodine supplement of around 150 micrograms per day. In addition, a daily dietary intake of 130 micrograms is advised. If your thyroid gland is not working properly you must first check with your doctor to see if it is safe for you to take extra iodine.

Vitamin D

Vitamin D, provided from dietary sources and sun exposure, is important for the growth of healthy bones. Australia has lots of sun and high rates of sun-damaged skin and skin cancers, including melanomas. Yet, many women cover up from the sun and have low vitamin D levels. They need to take supplements in pregnancy, especially during the winter months.

Probiotics

Probiotics have a potential protective role in maternal inflammatory and immune responses during pregnancy. The benefit of giving pregnant women probiotic pills to combat an infection called group B streptococcal (GBS) infection is being researched. This is a bacterial infection which can make newborn babies very sick.

Probiotics are living microscopic organisms, sometimes as small as just one cell. When ingested they have been found in sufficient amounts to confer direct effects on bacteria. They can modify the effects of some toxins from pathogenic or disease-causing bacteria as well as attenuating the host's inflammatory response. All this means that probiotics are a good thing. They are added to milk formula for babies, given to children with autism and help gut recovery after episodes of diarrhoea.

Fish oil

Fish oil taken during pregnancy may be protective for the development of the brain and nervous system in your baby. Fish with high contents of omega-3 fatty acids include tuna, salmon, mackerel, sardines, herring and trout.

Fish such as swordfish, marlin, shark (flake), sea perch and catfish are high in mercury content. Their intake should be limited during pregnancy. Other fish, including tinned tuna, are safer to eat.

Fish oil supplements contain the omega-3 fatty acids eicosapentaenoic acid (EPA) and docosahexaenoic acid (DHA). A daily dose of around 2 grams of fish oil is suggested.

What's not good for your baby?

Parental Duty

It is your responsibility to consider what is harmful for your baby. You may have to change your behaviour. You bear a parental duty of care for your unborn child.

Teratogens

Teratogens are agents that damage your unborn child – radiation, chemicals and drugs. Thalidomide was a drug prescribed in the 1950s and 1960s to reduce morning sickness. It caused the death of developing foetuses and severe limb damage to those babies born alive.

Isotretinoin (Roaccutane®) treats severe cystic acne. Its molecular structure resembles retinoic acid, a natural form of vitamin A. This plays a crucial role in embryonic development. Isotretinoin can damage the foetus. It is contraindicated in pregnancy and not given for at least a month prior to planning a pregnancy. The Australian Government Department of Health Therapeutic Goods Administration (TGA) provides online resources relating to the safe use of drugs during pregnancy and lactation. The safest practice remains no drugs, and caution with herbal and online preparations.

Alcohol

Any alcohol at any time during pregnancy is toxic to your unborn baby. A zero alcohol level is the only safe threshold. Foetal alcohol spectrum disorders (FASD) can result from prenatal exposure of the foetus to alcohol. Alcohol consumption during the first trimester (first 13 weeks) can result in face, organ and brain anomalies. In the second trimester there is a greater risk of spontaneous abortion, and in the third, an effect on body weight and size and brain growth.

Postnatal and later childhood neurobehavioural effects are common and include ADHD. Identified brain damage from FASD has implications within our justice system in terms of the competency of children, adolescents and young adults to provide reliable testimony. This is an area of controversial discussion.

Tobacco

If you smoke, so does your baby. You give your baby an unhealthy environment. It affects their growth and lungs. They could have a greater chance of ADHD.

Substances of abuse

Illicit drugs include crystal methamphetamine (ice), cocaine, heroin, cannabis (marijuana) and prescribed benzodiazepines (diazepam or Valium). Individual effects are uncertain but can include premature labour, the placenta breaking away from the wall of the uterus (placental abruption), small babies, and brain and heart abnormalities. Brain changes such as decreased arousal, increased stress and attention difficulties can occur.

Babies born to a mother with a drug addiction develop withdrawal symptoms. Neonatal abstinence syndrome occurs in the days following delivery. Babies experience a high-pitched cry, tremors, jitteriness, seizures, feeding problems, diarrhoea, vomiting, sweating and an increased breathing rate.

Mothers who are victims of addiction because of their genetic and environmental vulnerability need compassion, support, appropriate professional treatment and scrupulous follow-up. They don't need judgement. They could be your future daughter or granddaughter.

Domestic violence

Physical, sexual and emotional forms of abuse impact on the mother, unborn child, infant, young child, adolescent and emerging adult. These effects are transgenerational. They are a significant contributor to developmental trauma in a child. The impact of domestic violence flows over into our schoolyards, workplaces, roads and hospitals.

Excessive stress

Constant worry can adversely affect maternal mental health. Depression and anxiety in a mother and even in a maternal or paternal grandmother may have a negative long-term impact on the mental health of the unborn child.

Extreme exercise

Some sports are not baby-friendly. Avoid them during pregnancy. Scuba diving, skydiving and contact sports have inherent and unpredictable risks. They could jeopardise your life and that of your baby. Horseriding and downhill skiing carry the risk of sustaining a serious fall. Skiing poses the problem of being in a relatively remote setting should you have a pregnancy complication. Young infants carried in their skiing parent's backpack at the snow have died from hypothermia. Babies in spas can get overheated.

Infections

Bacterial and viral infections passed from a mother to her baby during pregnancy or at birth can cause significant illness. Rarely, a baby or a mother can die from these congenital infections, called TORCH infections. This acronym stands for toxoplasmosis, other (syphilis), rubella, cytomegalovirus (CMV) and herpes simplex virus (HSV).

Human immunodeficiency virus (HIV) infection, listeria, Varicella zoster (chicken pox), pertussis (whooping cough) and Group B streptococcus (GBS) can also affect babies. Your doctor will screen for these in early pregnancy.

Zika virus from mosquitoes has recently been associated with microcephaly (small head) in babies born in Brazil.

Most babies are born healthy. But, if you have had unprotected sex with an unknown partner with a history of hepatitis, substance abuse or genital herpes, you are at greater risk of having been exposed to an STI. You need to have a confidential medical consultation with your obstetrician or doctor.

If you don't have a natural or vaccination-derived immunity to chicken pox, rubella and whooping cough, your baby is vulnerable to contract these infections during your pregnancy or in the neonatal period.

If you want to read more about these infections and what you can do to prevent them, you can refer to the appendix section on 'Infections that can make your baby sick'.

Genes can make mistakes

Screening for chromosomal abnormalities

Mothers worry about having a baby with Down syndrome. This occurs when a baby receives an extra copy of chromosome 21, sometimes referred to as Trisomy 21. This results in specific and recognised facial characteristics, heart defects and significant learning impairments.

Nuchal fold test

Antenatal detection is available early, between nine and thirteen weeks of pregnancy. This involves an ultrasound to check the amount of fluid under the skin at the back of the baby's neck, called the nuchal fold thickness. A maternal blood test is also done to detect levels of two hormones. These are human chorionic gonadotropin (hCG) and pregnancy-associated plasma protein (PAPP-A). This combined test has a detection rate for Down syndrome of around 87 per cent.

Blood tests

A recent privately available and expensive blood test with 99.5 per cent accuracy for the detection of Trisomy 21 (Down syndrome), is non-invasive prenatal testing (NIPT). A simple maternal blood test taken after nine weeks of pregnancy is analysed for DNA fragments from the baby with results available from twelve weeks of gestation.

Between fifteen and seventeen weeks of pregnancy, a maternal blood test screens for Down syndrome and neural tube defects. This is called the Triple Test. It checks the levels of alpha-fetoprotein (AFP), which can be high in neural tube defects and low in Down syndrome. It measures the levels of the hormones, unconjugated oestriol and hCG. In Down syndrome there are usually low levels of AFP and oestriol and high levels of hCG.

Ultrasounds

Routine screening ultrasounds are done early to confirm foetal viability or later, from eighteen to twenty weeks, as a 'routine structural' scan. A range of congenital defects can be detected on ultrasound, including deformities of the heart and diaphragm, cleft lip and palate variants, abnormal head size, extra digits and gender.

Invasive antenatal tests

More invasive testing is offered when screening tests indicate a chromosomal abnormality such as Down syndrome, Trisomy 13 (Patau syndrome) or Trisomy 18 (Edwards syndrome). Trisomy 13 and 18 are genetic conditions associated with severe intellectual and physical disability with resultant short life spans of days or weeks.

Chromosomal defects such as these can be detected by chorionic villus sampling (CVS) or amniocentesis.

In CVS, cells are sampled from the placenta by a needle aspiration under ultrasound guidance. This test carries a risk of miscarriage which is less than 1 per cent. An accredited expert does this test. It can be done from ten to twelve weeks of pregnancy.

Amniocentesis is the procedure which samples the amniotic fluid or 'water' surrounding the baby. It can be done from fifteen to eighteen weeks of gestation and carries a similar miscarriage risk. Although a low risk, it is real. If your intent as a family is to continue with an abnormal pregnancy, you need to consider this before going ahead with an invasive diagnostic test on your baby.

Teamwork

Parenting as a partnership

If you are a sole parent you are not alone. There will be supportive friends and family happy to help you prepare for parenthood. There are some essential tasks for all parents to do before they bring their newborn baby home.

Be practical when choosing prams, strollers, baby cots, baths and highchairs.

I can recall Saturdays spent cruising around the various baby shops, checking out prams and strollers, baby cots and change tables. I had my heart set on a classic, old-fashioned pram. My husband wanted a robust, well-engineered, safe and light model that you could throw into your boot and pull out unscathed. After making me put each of these models into my car boot we came away with the lightest and safest stroller available.

Cots

Choose one that is simple and safe with easy access to your baby. Adjustable bases provide two levels. This allows you to put your baby in the cot from the newborn period. Place them in the lower half of the cot. Don't tuck in the bottom edge of the sheet and blanket.

If it fits, initially position the baby's cot in your bedroom. Bassinets can be expensive and your baby soon outgrows them. Big babies can get hot in them, especially in the warm summer months. Strollers aren't the best or safest overnight sleeping option.

Change tables

Simple tables that fold away are transportable and well priced. It helps to have them at optimal height for you. This protects your back. Babies move, so don't leave them alone on the bed or nappy change table. A baby's fall from the distance of a metre, even onto carpet, can result in a depressed skull fracture. Babies have soft, malleable eggshell skulls.

Nappy bags

Be prepared when leaving home with a baby or toddler. Take nappies, baby wipes, a disposable garbage bag, milk supplies, tissues and toys. Remember food and drinks for accompanying children and yourself.

Baby baths

Don't rush to buy a formal baby bath. Your baby will outgrow this quickly. A laundry tub works just as well. Remember to keep your baby's nose and mouth above the waterline.

Highchairs

Make sure they are easy to clean, with streamlined edges. Choose a large tray that can be fitted and cleaned easily. This catches the falling food scraps.

Cleaning

When I raised my children we were still trying to provide our children with a sterile environment. Mothers are now instructed to rinse bottles and teats out with water to avoid dried milk residue building up and to simply wash them in hot soapy water. Babies and infants need some exposure to 'germs' so that their bodies can build immunity and be less at risk of developing an allergy. Once your baby is crawling, they meet lots of germs.

Smacking

Don't shake, smack or whack a baby, infant, young child, older child, adolescent or young adult. Shaken babies can die. Corporal punishment removes trust and respect from the relationship you have with a child. It is an offence to physically strike a child. It is also just plain wrong. Would you kick your cat or dog? Your answer will be 'No'. So, don't ever strike a child.

Car seats

Child restraints for vehicles must meet Australian safety standards. A rearward-facing car restraint should be bought and fitted before you take your baby home from hospital.

When working as a paediatrician at a private maternity hospital I often saw frazzled fathers trying to fit the new baby restraint in their vehicle in the hospital carpark before collecting their partner and baby. Do this job early.

If you have two cars, you should think about putting a baby seat in each. Buying a child restraint for a grandparent to use in their vehicle might also be a good idea.

Kidsafe Child Restraint Guidelines provide an online summary of National Guidelines for the various types and use of child restraints at different ages and stages.

Night feeds

Don't fall asleep in bed while breastfeeding. Get up at night and feed your baby in a comfortable chair. It is unsafe to let your baby sleep with you. They can suffocate and die. On rare occasions this has occurred in hospitals when an exhausted mother has fallen asleep with her child.

Sudden infant death syndrome (SIDS)

In the past this was referred to as 'cot death'. The sudden and unexplained death of a child under 12 months of age is a tragic event. As a prospective new parent the best way of minimising this risk is to sleep your baby on their back from day one on a firm mattress. Avoid placing soft pillows or toys in the cot with your baby.

'Tummy time' can help strengthen your baby's neck muscles. Do this during waking hours when you can directly observe your baby. Keep your baby's head and face uncovered.

A hat can make full grown babies too hot. Small, very premature babies need a hat to keep warm.

A no-smoking environment and a co-shared environment for the first six to twelve months can be protective. Co-sleeping is not recommended. It is important that a safe sleeping environment applies for day and night sleeps.

There is a free downloadable SIDS and Kids Safe Sleeping app available in English and other languages which outlines preventive measures for SIDS.

Stillbirth

Any parent who has lost a child before, during or after birth carries their anguish forever. Still Aware is an organisation that educates future parents to connect early with their unborn child and to count their baby's kicks as a guide to the health of their unborn baby.

Their mantra is to help prevent the tragic figure of 2,500 stillborn babies in Australia each year. More information is available on their website.

Time to have a baby

The clock is ticking

As your due date approaches you will feel increasingly tired. This is expected. Most women work until thirty-four or thirty-six weeks into their pregnancy. This leaves little time to rest and prepare for the enormous challenge of caring for a newborn child. As family groups have contracted, the opportunity to look after young children prior to having one of your own is limited.

Raising your baby is a new experience. Finish work earlier, by thirty weeks if you can. This allows time to develop a household routine which you can continue when your baby is born. Many professional women don't have a schedule for buying groceries, cooking, doing laundry and cleaning bathrooms and floors before childbirth. They are too busy or someone does it for them. Make time to plan how you are going to stay organised when you change your role from corporate worker, or free and single person, to mother.

> *I went into hospital to have my first child with a bag of disposable nappies, one singlet and a bodysuit. Reflecting on this oversight, I rang my mother who dutifully sent by express post a parcel of essential baby clothing from interstate. We had set up everything else at home but it hadn't really hit me until entering the maternity ward that we were having a healthy baby and that life was about to change.*

Attend some antenatal classes and visit the birth suites at your hospital. Some women choose to have a home birth. I can't comment on this choice because of my traditional medical background. I have a skewed view because of my bad experiences involving mothers and babies rushed in from home to the hospital when things went horribly wrong.

Budgeting for a baby

It can be very expensive setting up your home for a baby. Pre-loved baby furniture is okay. Change tables do not need to be a feature furniture piece. They need to be functional.

A simple fold-up table placed in the shower recess works well and is easy to discard when no longer required.

Ongoing costs include medical fees, clothes, linen, nappies, bottles, breast pumps, food and toys, as well as the usual household costs.

Childcare can be excruciatingly expensive, especially when your work hours are reduced or absent. Some mothers have to seek childcare during the first twelve months of their child's life for financial reasons or to fulfil the requirements of their vocation.

Workplaces aren't always accommodating to women. Hopefully, this can change.

Birth plans

You can't micromanage birth

Birth plans were often discussed when I was having my children. Babies can't read birth plans and neither can busy obstetricians. If I had made a written birth plan for my obstetrician, it would have said, 'I want a healthy baby and I trust you to deliver one for me. I understand that might not happen'. Orchestrating the delivery of your child sets you up for failure and anxiety. Birth is unpredictable. You need to adopt a flexible mindset when having a baby because you will need this as you raise your child.

As a working paediatrician I saw very few formal written birth plans. I think this reflected the good relationship between the obstetrician and their patients. Never underestimate the strength and benefit of this mutual respect.

Many women have healthy, thriving children because of the skills and experience of their obstetrician, however, when doctors deliver thousands of babies there will be times when things go wrong. When this occurs families and their doctors and midwives will grieve.

The process of medical indemnity which seeks to assign blame does not facilitate healing. It fails to ensure adequate financial support for a patient who has ongoing needs because of an adverse clinical outcome. Mostly the causes for medical error are complex and multifactorial. Doctors, paediatricians and midwives do make mistakes. So do parents. Processes are in place to minimise these risks.

Where have all the chocolates gone?

When I started private paediatric practice in the late 1990s, there were always boxes of chocolates littering the nursing station desks of maternity wards. It was an unwritten rule that when you had a baby, you left a box of chocolates as a thank you to the caring staff. This custom contributed to a congenial workspace. By the mid-2000s this practice had tapered off, together with the simple courtesy of saying 'please' and 'thank you'. Symbolically, the paucity of chocolate wrappers reflects the changing face of healthcare.

> *The night before my elective caesarean section I couldn't sleep. A midwife came into my room to do routine nursing observations, went out and then returned with a mug of hot chocolate and time for a chat. Her kindness and gift of time made a difference and is remembered.*

In the busyness of our health profession we need to take time to listen and talk to people. Technology and efficiency can't replace compassionate care, conversation and touch.

Flying with your baby on board

Parents may travel interstate with their newborn child to see family and new grandparents. There are flight regulations pertaining to pregnancy and the postnatal period.

Australia's domestic airlines have strict rules for the carriage of pregnant mothers on their respective websites.

There are additional restrictions for complicated or multiple pregnancies and for flights lasting more than four hours. Rules also apply to postpartum mothers and newborn infants.

International flights have the additional constraints of entry rules for respective overseas countries.

Baby steps

Step into childhood gently – you have a long journey

Some couples aren't able to conceive. They can become parents through the processes of adoption and surrogacy. There are fathers who are still to meet their children. Some people choose not to have children. Sometimes the decision to parent is regretted. But, I have never met a parent who would willingly give back their child.

Parents who care for a severely disabled child are often selfless and savagely protective. They give up their lives and livelihood to care for the needs of their child. They celebrate every milestone, however small.

When you have the gift of a 'normal' or very 'gifted' child, try not to be complacent or brag about the ease with which your child reaches each developmental stage. Mothers' groups can decline into competitive forums which preside over the attainment of these milestones. Consider the parent whose child has severe autism and may never say their name. For those parents the joy of a first smile, hug, sound, word or simple act of play will be treasured. It will help them survive the hard journey of parenting.

I respect the choice of those who choose not to parent. They bear the responsibility of scaffolding the life of a child. They can be a mentor, role model, neighbour or brother. What they do, say and think will have an impact on children.

DOs

Do

- prepare for motherhood – what an awesome privilege
- discover your strengths and weaknesses when you have a baby
- get rid of 'selfies' – there is no place for narcissism in family life
- watch favourite movies, read books and relax before children
- continue to work on your relationship with your partner and family

DON'Ts

Don't

- have a rigid mindset about pregnancy
- replace the joy of pregnancy with fear and doubt
- adopt unrealistic expectations of parenthood
- pretend that having a child doesn't make a difference to your life
- make parenthood a competition
- forget to ask for help when you need it

Part 3

The early years – 0 to 5 years

A child's behaviour has its origins not only in the attitudes, personality and intelligence of the parents, and the way they manage him, but also in many innate features in the child and his response to his environment.

The Normal Child – Ronald S. Illingworth

First moments

Having your baby on board

Those first moments when you hold your baby are private, emotive and overwhelming. When our first child was born I recall the awe of being able to hold, cuddle and love her without handing her back. It was the realisation that we were now a family.

Our daughter was born on a day when the media headlines were about the horrific massacre of thirty-five people at Port Arthur in Tasmania by a lone gunman. The 29th of April 1996 was the day when Australia became anxious. This led to John Howard, the Prime Minister at the time, introducing strict gun ownership laws into our country. On a day when a new life had entered the world, the theatre staff were talking about death, disaster and tragedy. Selfishly, I reminded everyone that a baby had just been born and that the day was about hope. When evil occurs in the world it has the ability to creep and erode positive life forces. We must not let this happen.

The first smile

A wise friend and paediatrician warned me that the first six weeks with your baby can be ordinary, but that once your baby smiles for the first time, life gets better. Being told to have a low level of expectation when bringing my baby home helped.

The same friend warned me that it was difficult for dads. They can feel excluded from child raising until their child walks, talks and interacts with them. I think that 'dad confidence' has improved over more recent years. Most dads are happy to have a go at practical parenting. This is a good thing.

As a new mother I found that I was playing catch–up with my child's development. I would achieve a good settling routine and then my child's behaviour would suddenly change. My paediatrician told me to 'go with the flow'. This laid–back approach was good advice.

Fatigue, anxiety and depression can overlap in the challenging first weeks of being home alone with a newborn baby. As extended families have contracted, many new mothers have had minimal contact with babies or young children. Holding their baby for the first time is strange or even frightening. They feel uncertain and inadequate.

New mothers need emotional and practical support. It is alright for them to set the rules about visiting times. To ask a friend to bring morning tea or a meal when they visit.

The routine tasks of caring for a baby are difficult for a mother, particularly if she is tired and used to taking charge. My challenge was bathing my first child. I found this a daunting task each day, until a friend, and sensible mother, told me to let my husband shower with our baby. She gave me permission to do a baby 'sponge bath' some days. Babies stay clean and cope with the occasional missed bath as long as you maintain good skin care, especially in the nappy area and skin creases.

The best thing about this advice was that my friend followed it up by changing a nappy or making me a cup of coffee.

My sister's advice was to never to disturb a sleeping baby. My amendment to this tip is unless they are sick as indicated by poor feeding, a fever, being too cold or overly sleepy. If your baby is floppy, lethargic, and pale or mottled in colour, they could be ill.

Social and academic boundaries offer little protection when it comes to bringing up children. Irrespective of our background, raising a child will be the most challenging and humbling experience of our lives.

If you are fortunate to have supportive family and friends, ask for help and show gratitude. People respond to being needed as long as there is reciprocal care and compassion. It can be difficult logistically when families are separated by state boundaries or ocean. However, there is air travel.

When I left Melbourne to commence work as a flying doctor in the Eastern Goldfields Section of the Royal Flying Doctor Service in Kalgoorlie, my father reassured me that home was just a plane ride away. Fast forward a few years and I was settled in Perth with my husband. I was raising two daughters and juggling a busy paediatric practice. There were several interstate 'plane rides' during that time, instigated by my father. He would phone and tell me that my mother was coming to stay for a couple of weeks. I would never ask, but he would always know when she was needed.

Even if you are a 'professional', you are still just another mum or dad. You don't have to be the best parent in the street. You are already the best parent for your child. Raising children is not a competition.

I remember one morning trying to get my toddler secured in her car seat so we could get out of the house. After multiple false starts due to a number of bodily functions firing off at rapid rate, I decided to just drive and deal with the mess later. I'm glad I did, because we ended up having a fun day, even though I left the stroller behind in the driveway.

Just give parenting a go. Be prepared to listen to advice along the way. Change your previous ideas, or those of your family, relating to the care of a child. This is important when you have a child with physical, emotional or social challenges. Having a child with autism incorporates many of these challenges. It requires great patience, compassion, understanding, hope and lots of help.

Parenthood necessitates that for a time you focus less on self and more on family.

Maintain a cool and calm façade. Raising a child is not the time to be perfect. It is not about having flawless nails, well-behaved hair or immaculate make-up. For some women this is important. Their looks or career define who they are and allow them to function best as a mum. Don't judge those few 'super-mums'. They are good mums as long as they can maintain the balance. When you meet them just try not to look jealous! Acknowledge their competency. Learn some tips from them. They usually have great organisational skills.

One of my friends always had the perfect picnic basket with prepared baby meals in small plastic containers, labelled drink bottles and cut-up fruit. I was always grateful to have remembered to bring my children and turn up at the right place and time! If I forgot the food I would buy some at a nearby café.

My hero was a paediatric colleague with several young children. On a picnic to Perth's Kings Park she just took a bag of sliced bread. She handed this out to her kids. This served the dual purpose of addressing their hunger and feeding the ducks. She took home happy, active but tired and only slightly hungry children. A perfect play day!

The first six weeks

Early days

The postnatal period encompasses the first four to six weeks after you deliver your baby. Most hospitals aim to get the mother and baby home as quickly as possible following a normal pregnancy and delivery. This has the benefit of infection control and engaging a new mother with community services as early as possible.

Within the private sector the postnatal stay tends to be longer, particularly if women have had a caesarean section. This time is used to establish breastfeeding and parent-crafting skills such as handling, bathing and changing nappies.

A resource-rich environment with caring midwives assists the successful establishment of breastfeeding. This confers the benefits of bonding, cheap nutrition and immune protection. It is also a protective factor for SIDS.

A paediatric colleague once told me that breastfeeding was either easy or hard – there was no in-between. I think she was right. I have listened to women express guilt over their inability or failure to breastfeed. I might be seeing a 15 year old and a guilt-ridden mother will say, 'I only breastfed for three weeks'.

Some mothers are unable to breastfeed because of illness, medications or insufficient supply. A good midwife recognises when to change the slogan from 'breastfeed or bust' to 'fed is best'. You can bottle-feed your baby and still bond with them. Milk formula is not a sin. There are many types of milk formula. But, if you give your baby a goat milk formula, check that it has added folate. Natural goat milk is too low in folate for babies.

Bonding with your baby is not solely determined by whether you breastfeed or not. You can still have skin-to-skin contact or 'kangaroo care' with your term or preterm infant when you bottle-feed. Guilt has a busy enough job, without burdening mothers who can't or decide not to breastfeed.

Breastfeeding problems
When I have asked about the developmental history of their child, mothers will lament that they couldn't breastfeed their baby. Even a drop of colostrum, which precedes the flow of breastmilk, is a good start for your baby. There will be harder battles ahead than whether you breastfed or not.

Some mothers will find breastfeeding painful. If their baby attaches poorly at the breast, the nipples can become cracked and bleed. Breast engorgement is uncomfortable and can lead to mastitis or breast infection. This can rapidly make a mother ill.

If you develop a high temperature with muscle aches and pains, chills and shakes and have redness and pain in your breast, you need to be seen by a doctor. Antibiotics taken by mouth or given in a drip in hospital will be required. Still express and retain your breastmilk supply.

Thrush around the nipples, passed back and forwards from your breast and baby's mouth, can also cause severe pain. I told you that breastfeeding was either easy or hard!

Early feeding

Talk with your child health nurse about the best time to start solids for your baby. Usually this is around four to six months. Babies need to chew textured and lumpy foods to develop strong muscles in the mouth. This is important for speech production. Good head control helps. To develop this, babies require some time spent prone, known as 'tummy time'.

Other 'stuv' – settling, sleeping, tummy upsets and vomiting

All babies are different. That is why there are so many books on how to settle and feed them. If you are struggling with your 3-week-old baby, ask for help from the child health nurse, local doctor, family, neighbours and friends. Eventually, your baby will outgrow these common problems.

Babies from 3 weeks to 3 months have 'colic' and 'wind'. We don't know what causes this, but it goes away. If it doesn't, your baby may have an inflammation of their stomach lining, called gastritis, due to gastro-oesophageal reflux. Stomach acid burns and hurts. Babies scream because they are in pain. They also vomit.

Lactose intolerance from milk can upset your baby's stomach and gut. They have frothy stools which burn their bottom. They can pass blood.

Vomiting can be a medical problem such as reflux. Urine infections, blood sepsis and meningitis can cause vomiting. So do viral infections such as 'gastro'. You will need a doctor to sort out persistent vomiting problems.

Surgical blockages cause vomiting, usually with green bile. Restriction of the stomach outlet is a condition called pyloric stenosis. If your baby has this, they will have forceful or projectile vomits, lose weight and become unwell. This presents early, before 3 months.

A blockage of the fluid around the brain causes hydrocephalus. Babies with this have a rapid increase in head circumference and vomit.

Intussusception occurs when one portion of the bowel telescopes into an adjacent part. Your baby or young child may first be diagnosed with simple gastroenteritis, but then become rapidly ill. This condition is seen most in children from 3 months to 6 years of age.

Child health nurse visits

When you leave the protective walls of the hospital you are not alone. Community child health centres provide care for babies and young children up to the age of 4 years. An assigned child health nurse will receive notification of all newborn babies in their area and contact you to do an early baby visit. If English is not your first language, your child health nurse can visit with an interpreter. For some socially isolated women, this provides a rare chance to speak freely with another person.

The first visit may be in your home. Valuable and helpful observations are made at this visit. The child health nurse can be the first person to detect postnatal depression symptoms. They support mothers to raise resilient children. Their role is pivotal in the early recognition and prevention of significant mental and physical health problems in young children and families.

At a book club meeting we were reminiscing about the impact of the child health nurse visit to our homes when our babies were just a few weeks old. The recollections were of reverence for the care, reassurance and competency of an experienced nurse to walk us through those difficult times. Our children are now teenagers or young adults. That tells you something about the value of experienced child health nurses.

A jaundiced view of life

About 60 per cent of newborn babies look yellow. This is called jaundice. It first appears in the eyes and then the skin. Mostly this is normal. It appears after twenty-four hours and is gone within two to three weeks. It can last for six weeks. This is called physiological jaundice. Jaundice which occurs in the first twenty-four hours or persists after six weeks is abnormal. It is called pathological jaundice.

Serious bacterial infections can cause jaundice. So can haemolysis or rapid breakdown of red blood cells. This can occur when a mother has a particular type of blood group and her baby has another. These conditions include ABO incompatibility and Rh isoimmunisation. Babies affected by these conditions in utero can become very anaemic. Your obstetrician will let you know if you are at risk and will check your blood group during early pregnancy.

If your baby looks yellow make sure they are checked by a midwife, child health nurse, local doctor or paediatrician. Most paediatricians who see your baby in hospital will follow them up in their rooms at 6 weeks. If your baby is very jaundiced, sleepy and not feeding before this, check to see if you will need to see someone sooner. Is your baby getting enough milk? Do they have an infection, thyroid problem or other medical condition?

There is more information about jaundice in the reference, and resources section of this book.

More tests

Newborn screening tests

All newborn babies are screened for diseases that if undetected and untreated can cause significant physical disability, intellectual disability or death. Blood is taken from the baby's heel with a skin-prick test called the 'Guthrie test'. This is done when the baby is 3 to 5 days of age and after they have commenced oral feeding. The baby's blood is collected on a blotting paper card. You will be notified if your baby has an abnormal Guthrie result.

Phenylketonuria (PKU), congenital hypothyroidism, galacto-saemia, cystic fibrosis and rare metabolic disorders can be detected and treated early.

Congenital hypothyroidism means that a baby doesn't make enough thyroid hormone. There are a number of causes for this condition which may be transient. Early and urgent treatment prevents problems with brain development. Around 1 in 2,000 to 1 in 4,000 babies have this disorder

Methylmalonic acidaemia (MMA) is a rare inherited organic acid disorder that is screened for on the Guthrie. In this disorder, certain proteins and fats (lipids) can't be broken down and utilised properly. When an affected person is stressed, such as having an acute illness, they can develop life-threatening problems because of low blood sugar levels.

About 80 per cent of rare conditions are genetic in origin. A number of support groups provide an advocacy role for children and families who have to cope with rare diseases. They include Unique, understanding chromosome disorders, based in the UK; Rare Voices Australia; and Australian Rare Chromosome Awareness Network (ARCAN). Western Australia also runs the Genetic and Rare Disease Network (GaRDN).

Further information is available on their websites and is referenced in this book.

Babies need to hear

One to two babies in 1,000 are reported to be born with hearing loss in both ears. Newborn hearing screening tests are now widely available. Testing can be done from 6 hours of age until 3 months. I recommend that you have your baby tested during the postnatal period. Early intervention in a child with a hearing deficit makes a difference. Good hearing is imperative for language development.

Close ties

Maternal and child bonding

The bond that develops between a mother and her child is shown in the 'Still Face' experiment. This was presented at a conference in 1975 by Edward Tronick, a developmental psychologist from Harvard University. You can search for this and watch it online.

The experiment demonstrates the powerful visual image of a mother engaging socially with her 12-month-old baby. The mother then turns away. She adopts an expressionless face. The child tries to re-engage her with squeals, claps and hand gestures. Soon the baby becomes visibly upset, withdraws and cries. The distressed mother then provides comfort and reassurance to her child. This demonstration shifted prior thinking that somehow babies lacked the emotion that we feel as adults and were unable to respond to their environment.

A secure early attachment is protective for children. It builds emotional resilience. This helps children develop into strong and happy adolescents and young adults.

The child who experiences developmental trauma from emotional, physical and sexual abuse or neglect sustains long-term adverse social, emotional and cognitive consequences. That is why it is so important that the baby, infant and young child's brain is wired securely.

Attachment

Dr John Bowlby was a significant psychiatrist and 'the father of attachment theory'. His book *A Secure Base,* published in 1988, talks about the integral role of effective parenting and secure early childhood attachments. He made the logical statement: 'To be a successful parent means a lot of very hard work'. Perhaps he even sensed the social change that bred narcissistic parenting when he said, 'Giving time and attention to children means sacrificing other interests and activities'.

He acknowledged the pivotal early work of Mary Ainsworth, an American-Canadian developmental psychologist, on the different types of attachment behaviour displayed by a child when placed in a stressful situation with a caregiver. These studies, designed in 1965, were known as the Strange Situation Procedure. The observed response of a child with their caregiver and that with a stranger indicated the level of the child's emotional resilience and ability to communicate, self-regulate and deal with stress. It was felt to reflect the level of security in the child's attachment with their parent.

It is essential that newborn babies are exposed to the sensory richness of their surrounds. They need visual, olfactory and tactile stimulation as well as feed time, quiet time and rest. It is incredulous that the healing effect of maternal touch for the agitated crying baby took science so long to confirm. Some of the studies on maternal and infant bonding and the importance of the socialisation of the newborn infant, such as those by Klaus and Kennell, only started appearing during the 1980s. If someone had bothered to speak with mothers earlier they would know how important it is to touch, talk, sing, watch and comfort your baby and child.

Oxytocin

Early maternal–infant interaction is very powerful. It can be measured by physiological and biological markers such as maternal oxytocin levels. This hormone is released in pulsatile bursts from a special endocrine gland situated in our brain, called the pituitary gland. This occurs when mothers breastfeed. Oxytocin is measured at more sustained levels in response to the positive social and emotional responses that are created between a mother and her newborn child.

Most babies will bond to one carer, generally their mother, within the first month of life. This bonding link is very important as correlated by raised oxytocin levels.

The potential for oxytocin levels to rise in situations where empathy, closeness and trust abound has led to some people trialling oxytocin as a nasal spray for children with autism. This is not a cure for autism. Intensive social and behavioural support must still be provided to build the social strengths of the child.

Parental mental health

Postnatal depression and high anxiety affect a mother. Parents with postnatal depression struggle to provide positive social messages to their baby.

Our mental health services provide valuable early intervention to prevent and address disordered maternal and infant attachment. Timely, targeted programs to secure attachment between a parent and child include the 'Circle of Security'. Parents can further research this online, but are best to discuss it with their child health nurse or other healthcare professional.

All states and territories have infant and child support services to assist families with the complexity of early child raising. These include Ngala and Ngala DadsWA in Western Australia, Tresillian Family Care Centres in New South Wales and Tweddle Child and Family Health Service and Parentline in Victoria.

Many states, in recognition of the importance of the father's role in effective parenting and positive child outcome, have targeted 'lad friendly' antenatal parenting programs which take place in the local pub. These include 'Beer and Bubs' and 'mr. dad' initiatives. It's where blokes talk to blokes who have survived the first weeks at home with a newborn baby. If you are a high-achieving perfectionist dad, attendance should be compulsory.

Child rearing demands freedom. If you are a dad or co-parent, you can't hold your partner's hand all the time. Support them, but don't suffocate them during this early child-raising period. There is sufficient time to bond with your baby. You will be better primed to do this if you have some sleep reserve when your baby and partner come home from hospital.

Don't appear too self-sufficient when you have a baby. Ask for all the help you can get. When people visit you at home suggest that they come with a fruit and cheese platter or cake for morning tea. Babies and illness are times when you need practical help from the village.

If you are not the child-bearing parent, never misconstrue the validity and place of your parenting role. This applies in all relationships, including same-sex, adoptive and surrogate. Every parent and carer is important.

Life through childhood SPECS

Early childhood development

SPECS encompasses all of the early childhood developmental stages: *S*peech, language and communication; *P*hysical fitness, fine and gross motor coordination; *E*motional resilience; *C*ognitive growth; and *S*ocial competency. These essential milestones provide the strong foundations for children to grow into healthy adults.

Social smiles

A baby looks at the way a sound is made by observing the different shapes the lips make when producing that sound. They hear the sound coming from the lips and start to understand connections between sounds and their assigned objects. Infants listen and respond to the emotion of the sound. The child matches the social signs for happy with a laugh or chuckle, and harsh, angry sounds with a furrowed face. They learn to perform for the reassurance of their mother's smile and her warm caress. When a mother is depressed, tired or stressed, her emotions alter. She can appear cold and distant. The baby becomes confused and then unsettled, irritable and withdrawn. They cry. Don't panic if your baby cries. This can be normal. It is the way they communicate and learn. It takes time for a mother to learn their language.

Babies start to mimic facial expressions from the moment they are born. Babies will demonstrate a smile with a grimace or protrude a tongue during this brief period of heightened alertness. Whilst it is 'normal' for a first smile to be recorded at around 6 to 8 weeks of age, some babies develop a social smile much earlier. The difference between a reflex or 'windy' smile and a real smile is the emotional content of the smile. A social smile is the way a baby communicates pleasure with another person.

> *I attended the delivery of one baby, a little boy. He was very alert at birth. When I saw him later on the maternity ward with his mother, he gave me a smile. He was just 2 days old. 'Did you see that?' I asked his mother. 'Yes', she said. 'I thought I had just imagined it, but he smiled at me too'.*

Don't panic if your baby is not smiling until 10 weeks. This can be normal. Some babies have a delay with visual maturation and just take longer. However, it is reassuring for your baby to be smiling by 8 weeks.

Hearing and vision

Mothers 'feel' their baby respond to sound during pregnancy. It is reassuring when newborn hearing screens confirm that their baby can hear.

The development of vision and hearing have early critical windows of optimal development. The brain needs to get visual and auditory signals very early so that it can make sense of these messages and interpret them as pictures and sounds. Babies move their eyes in unison by 6 months. Visual messages are processed in the visual cortex of the brain, an area in the occipital or rear part of the brain. This is why if you fall and strike the back of your head you 'see stars'.

Squints

If the infant brain does not receive the correct visual signals because of a severe squint, or if a baby is born with a cataract that covers the lens of their eye, the brain won't be able to interpret the pictures it is seeing. That is why it is important to identify squints very early and have them assessed medically. If a squint is confirmed your baby has to see a paediatric ophthalmologist (eye doctor) for treatment.

It can be helpful to keep 'red eye' blemishes on your baby's photo or digital image. If the red eye reflex is not the same in each eye, your baby may have a squint. A white reflex could indicate a serious problem. Squints that come and go are not as serious as fixed ones. They still have to be checked out.

Management of a confirmed squint involves patching the baby's good eye. This forces the 'weak' eye to see. Eye drops produce the same effect by dilating the pupil of the baby's good eye. This blurs the vision and forces the baby to focus with their weak eye.

Some babies have abnormal eye movements that are undetected in the newborn period. Nystagmus consists of circular or rotatory eye movements and needs to be investigated by a paediatric ophthalmologist.

'Glue ear'

Hearing and vision are screened at the time of school entry when a child is around 5 years of age.

One of the most common causes of childhood hearing loss and early language delay is the chronic inflammatory ear condition, known as 'glue ear' or 'fluid in the ear'. If this is detected, a referral to an ENT surgeon by your local doctor or paediatrician is required.

Treatment of glue ear involves the surgical procedure of draining the fluid from the middle ear space with a small plastic tube called a grommet or ventilation tube. This is inserted through a small incision made in the eardrum by the surgeon. Your child is asleep under a general anaesthetic and won't be in pain. The tympanic membrane (eardrum) heals behind the grommet tube. Doctors and researchers are starting to look at ways of assisting the child's immune system to tackle the problem of chronic glue ear.

While a child is waiting for surgery they don't hear sounds clearly. They lose valuable language learning time. The child whose hearing loss is reversed after having grommets inserted can show a dramatic improvement in their behaviour and language. This is a wonderful transformation for parents, teachers, speech pathologists and paediatricians to witness.

Upon school entry the child with poor hearing discrimination due to 'fluid in the ear' can present as 'naughty' or inattentive. Inappropriate diagnoses of ADHD, learning and language disorders, sensory processing problems, auditory processing disorders and autism can be assigned to a child who just can't hear.

Hearing screens
All states and territories have excellent private and public services that can assess hearing. Referral can be made by a child health nurse, doctor or parent.

Protect hearing
We need to introduce better policies and preventive measures to care for our children's hearing. We connect our kids to electronic noise at close range through earpieces from a young age. During the adolescent years we fail to enforce the wearing of earplugs

when they work in noisy workplace environments such as bars and nightclubs.

Noise exposure in young children is a potential public health issue. It affects the capacity of our future adults to hear. Noise-attenuating earmuffs could have a role for children.

As you lose the capacity to discriminate the difference between the sound of 'b' and 'd' or 'v' and 't' in conversation, or when the sound of normal conversational speech becomes distorted in a noisy room, you begin to feel socially isolated, frustrated and even depressed.

Speech and language

Before babies communicate with words they will use their cries and screams. Toddlers and young children will have physical outbursts – emotional meltdowns and temper tantrums. They are normal unless extreme, persistent or a disproportionate reaction.

Parents and early childhood educators have to learn this language so that they can communicate with a child without overreacting.

By 8 weeks, babies will search for sound with their eyes. They are unable to localise it until closer to 5 months. At this age they will turn their head towards a sound.

First sounds

Babies will settle from 5 to 6 months when they hear soothing music. They talk in 'babble' to other people. It is very important to listen to what they are saying and to respond with proper words and speech. We are not babies, so we shouldn't speak like them.

Babies respond when called from 7 months. They generally know their name by 13 to 14 months.

Babies will blow raspberries and make blurting, explosive sounds around 6 to 9 months.

By 9 months, babies have developed some babbled phrases and can say 'mum, mum' or 'dad, dad'. Usually they say 'dad, dad' first. This is a very wise choice for a baby!

Early memory

Children love the game peek-a-boo from 10 to 12 months of age. This milestone coincides with the development of early visual memory and is referred to as 'the awareness of object permanence'. It is a pivotal cognitive stage in development. It heralds the emergence of the child from the toddler, a person who shakes their head for 'no', and means it.

From 11 months baby talk consists of self-babble with two to three words emerging by 12 months of age.

Action and anticipatory games such as 'peek-a-boo' and 'round and round the garden, like a teddy bear' are important interactive social and language games. They are enjoyed from 10 to 12 months.

Sentences

There is great variability in the acquisition of language between 12 and 20 months and it can all be normal. A child will usually have four to ten words at 15 months and twenty words at 20 months.

A child needs around forty words before they have a sufficient vocabulary to join two words together. This occurs around the age of 2 years. It is reassuring if your child has five two-word combinations at this age. They will start to repeat words constantly, known as echolalia. This will drive you nuts. Children also start to use pronouns such as 'I' and 'me'.

Language acquisition is exponential. By 2.5 years, children have a vocabulary of more than two hundred words. Self-talk and imaginative play emerges. They ask, 'What?', 'Why?' and 'Who?' Parents must find the patience to answer these questions. This is how children learn.

By the end of the third year, a child speaks well in sentences of six or more syllables such as, 'I want to go to the park'.

Pre-literacy skills

It is vital that a child is exposed to a rich word and language environment in the first three years of their life. This improves their vocabulary and contributes to their early IQ scores. Children also require digital literacy, but parents should monitor the appropriate use of electronic screens.

Children's TV programs such as *Play School, Dora the Explorer* and *Sesame Street* promote language, but others don't. Parents need to take charge of what their young child views.

A child raised in a home which has no books and treats literacy with neglect will struggle to embrace reading. Children who are encouraged to read are already ahead socially, emotionally and academically when they start school. It is very hard to catch up the deficit of vocabulary accrued in the early years.

All children love sharing familiar stories from books. Make sure you choose books that you enjoy. You will read them a lot!

Children need exposure to pre-literacy material during the first three to four years of life. Mem Fox's *Giraffe in the Bath, Baby Bedtime* and *Where Is the Green Sheep?* and the Dr Seuss series are excellent children's books. They have a strong emphasis on rhyme and phonics, making them excellent resources. I have listed a number of children's book in the bibliography section.

Think about how you can create a rich pre-literacy environment for your child with a balance of tactile and electronic books, talking books, music and toys. Ask other parents what books and toys their children like.

A degree in law, commerce, engineering, medicine or education won't help you with a decision about which book or toy is best for your baby. Parenthood is a very humbling experience. You might have to ask for help, even from your own mum or your partner's mother!

Language and cognitive growth

The behaviour of the young child is the way they communicate. Play is a child's internal language. Parents can understand their child better when they learn this.

The 2-year-old child who does not talk, but plays imaginatively and with purpose, will likely develop language.

Everyone will tell you about the child who did not talk until they were 24 months, but then spoke in full sentences. These children understand language commands, are competent with role-play and undertake complex symbolic play. They don't have autism.

The amazing reality of child development is the exponential gain of vocabulary and use of increasingly inferential language as a child grows. This is most impressive from the age of 3 years and 9 months. The terrible twos and the tumultuous threes disappear. Children start to have conversations, try out new words and by 4 years of age they can lie.

They start to choose friends, share and participate in group play. Young children enjoy dress-ups and role-model play. They regulate their emotions more because they can communicate with words.

4 year olds

The brain of the 4-year-old child is evolving and developing. They hope and dream. Fears of the dark and nightmares emerge.

Some children have 'night terrors'. They are a part of normal childhood development, can run in families and are not harmful to your child. 'Night terrors' occur in deep sleep with an onset around 2 to 3 years of age, lessening as later childhood and adolescence approaches. You will recognise if your child has one of these. They will scream or cry out, look frightened, with eyes wide open but go back to sleep with no recollection of the event in the morning.

The 4-year-old child yearns for some sense of control and early independence. This can be a fine balance, but remember that you are the adult and the parent. You are not the playmate and friend. Embed this in your memory for when your child becomes an adolescent.

Kindergarten

Kindergarten children enjoy exploring outdoors, social events and activities. One of the traps of having so many choices is that young children are used to being entertained. They will often ask, 'What are we doing now?' Sometimes you need to challenge them and ask, 'What are you going to do – it's free play time'.

Children have to learn to construct play out of nothing. Not many kids can do this. Ask your child, 'What do you do for fun?'

Articulation errors

'Normal' children can have problems with the 'r', 't', 'f' and 'th' sounds. Help from a speech pathologist ensures they have resolved around the age of 4 years. The 's' sound takes a little longer, up to the age of 5 to 6 years, to get right.

Lisps and stutters can start around 2 to 4 years. Many children will work out stutters and get rid of them by 6 years. Not all kids can do this. It is best to have your child checked and monitored by a speech pathologist.

One method of managing stutters is the Lidcombe Program. This uses positive verbal feedback when your child doesn't stutter. Your child is not stuttering on purpose or being lazy with their speech.

5 year olds

At 5 years of age, a child's grammar and fluency has greatly improved. The 's-f-th' group of phonetic sounds can remain problematic for kids until between the ages of 4 and 6, even with speech pathology input. Jokes become very popular. Children of this age devour stories and will act them out.

Make time for bedtime stories as a fun routine and not as a chore. If your child sees you rolling your eyes and yawning at this time, they will soon learn that reading isn't fun. You should be racing your partner to your child's bedside in the hope that you will get the privilege of reading alongside them.

Physical development

Gross motor milestones

Babies move sequentially from wiggling and squirming to flipping, turning and crawling. Most babies will crawl before they grab onto a bit of furniture and pull themselves up to stand. Some babies sit for a while, ponder and then one day decide to stand up.

Babies should kick well by 3 months. They kick before they are born. You can feel and see this. From birth, babies can lift their heels up from the change table. If they don't, they could have a hip, muscle or nerve problem.

Spinal muscular atrophy

One of the most devastating neuromuscular (muscles, nerves and spinal cord) conditions is spinal muscular atrophy (SMA). This is a genetic disorder which occurs when affected genes are passed to a child from both the mother and father. It usually presents in the first 3 to 12 months of life. Specialised nerve cells in the spinal cord aren't programmed properly to send messages to muscle cells. A child will have extreme weakness in the distal muscles of their arms and legs, as well as the muscles in their diaphragm and chest wall.

There are four types of this disease, with the infantile form being particularly severe. Children die within the first two years of life. Fortunately, it is rare.

I saw a child in her first year of life who presented as always being chesty, with a weak cough. She was floppy and not able to kick her legs when her nappy was changed. This infant was alert, happy and socially engaging. I still carry the sadness I felt for this child and her loving family when I saw the small muscle tremors in her tongue, called fasciculations – a pathognomonic sign of this terrible disease.

If this disease is suspected, a child needs urgent referral to a paediatric neurologist or to be seen at a children's hospital.

Further details of this condition are well documented on the Spinal Muscular Atrophy (SMA) Australia website.

First steps

Babies start to roll from their back to their stomach by 7 to 8 months and will be trying to crawl. From 10 to 11 months they begin to pull themselves up to stand by holding onto furniture. Babies have to weight-bear. Too many sit propped up in strollers and highchairs. They need 'tummy time' and 'crawl time' to grow strong legs.

First steps can be as early as 8 to 9 months, but usually occur at 11 to 15 months. If you have a family history of late walkers, don't expect your baby to walk early.

If your child is not walking by 20 to 22 months, they should have some screening tests. These tests include an X-ray of the hips to make sure the hips are not dislocated, a thyroid function test and a creatine kinase (CK) level test. CK is a muscle enzyme which can be extremely high in serious muscle and neurological disorders.

Hip problems

Check with family about any history of dislocated hip problems, known as developmental dysplasia of the hip (DDH). This can cause a problem with walking if not detected early. Girls, first-born babies and those delivered breech (bottom first) are more likely to have DDH.

Picked up early, DDH is generally corrected by an abduction splint. This device is put on under the nappy to keep the legs apart in a frog like position. An orthopaedic doctor will follow your baby's hip growth if one or both are completely or partially dislocated.

Most cases of DDH are picked up at the newborn examination by a midwife, local doctor, or paediatrician. If you have a family history of DDH or if your baby is born breech, make sure that you tell your doctor so that they can arrange a screening ultrasound in the first four weeks after birth.

Jumping

At 15 months your baby crawls up the stairs. They have enough strength in their thighs to jump from a flat surface by 20 to 24 months.

The child who demonstrates the 'Gowers' sign' – needs to hold onto their legs to assist them in rising from sitting to standing – has significant weakness. They can't jump. They may have a serious muscle disorder.

Duchenne muscular dystrophy

The two main muscle disorders are Duchenne muscular dystrophy and a milder form Becker muscular dystrophy. These diagnoses are confirmed by a high level of the muscle enzyme CK and a muscle biopsy.

Children who have big but weak calf muscles and are not jumping by 2 years may have the genetic neuromuscular disorder of Duchenne muscular dystrophy. This affects mostly boys with an incidence of around 1 in 3,500 boys born worldwide. Further information relating to this disorder and its management are available on the Muscular Dystrophy Australia website.

Hopping

The 3-year-old child stands on one leg briefly, walks on tiptoes and goes upstairs with just one foot on each step. At around 4 to 5 years of age they can confidently walk downstairs like an adult, but will still need to put both feet on each step.

The 4-year-old child should be able to jump from a step, ride a tricycle, hop and climb ladders and trees. Many 4 year olds can't do this, because we overprotect them. How many kids do you see swinging from trees?

Ball skills require practice. Kids don't get enough time or space to throw and catch a ball or hit a ball with a bat. Backyards have contracted and home media rooms have expanded.

Skipping, hopping, dancing, throwing, batting and catching are all skills achievable by the 5-year-old child if given the opportunity to develop them.

Schools complain that kids come to school unable to hop, skip or jump. There used to be a game called hopscotch. Most young kids can't play this today. They don't have well-developed gross motor skills.

Schools are introducing programs to promote physical fitness. They are suggesting games in which kids jump like a kangaroo or crawl like a crocodile.

Electronic games have a role and are good fun, but they don't replace the physicality of outdoor activities.

School sport teachers are concerned about the drop in physical fitness and increase in obesity in young kids. Children must swim with confidence in a country surrounded by water.

Teaching your child to swim is a mandatory life skill. It is your responsibility as a parent to make sure your child can do this.

Funny feet

Check your baby's feet. If the posture of your newborn child's foot is abnormal and not corrected by passive stretching of the foot, you will need an orthopaedic doctor to have a look at your baby's foot. Do this early.

Most funny-looking feet are normal. Your baby's feet have probably been in a cramped position during your pregnancy and need time to unfold on their own. Babies born in the breech position often have 'squashed-looking' feet.

Some familial and genetic conditions affect feet. Abnormally prominent high arches (pes cavus), if progressive with growth through childhood, can be problematic. Some uncommon neurological conditions such as Charcot–Marie–Tooth are characterised by high arches, weak feet and foot drop. They require a paediatric neurologist and orthopaedic surgeon opinion.

Babies change their brain

Neuroplasticity

Neuroplasticity is a term often seen in the media. It refers to the potential for the brain to reroute its neural circuitry after injury, such as stroke. We are learning that this can occur at all stages of life.

When I was working as a neonatal registrar, I looked after a lot of premature babies. Some of these babies had major abnormalities on their early brain ultrasounds and head scans due to bleeding in the brain. Yet, they were moving, feeding and responsive. Many of these changes resolved. Even when residual brain changes were seen on brain images, you wouldn't always see the consequences of these in the child. Some babies were not so fortunate and suffered residual physical and intellectual deficits such as muscle weakness, stiff limbs, vision and hearing problems, and learning and intellectual difficulties.

If you are the parent of a child with a disability, don't focus on what their brain can't do. Think about what it can and might do.

Cerebral palsy

Cerebral palsy is a non-progressive physical condition which occurs before, during or after birth. It can change in presentation as a child grows and affects movement and posture by its impact on muscles and the way they move. It can be mild, affecting just a hand, or severe, affecting the whole body, including muscles used for swallowing, seeing and talking. Cerebral palsy affects around 2 per 1,000 live births.

There is exciting research in this area. Innovative and intensive physical therapy programs have an increasing clinical role. Serial plaster casting and Botox injections are used to help relax tight muscles that are impeding function.

Children with diagnosed cerebral palsy benefit from the research and new methods of intensive rehabilitation intervention implemented through tertiary children's hospitals and allied services.

Wonky walks

Beware the child who limps

If you sit in a shopping centre, you will notice an extraordinary array of gaits (walks). Not many will be 'normal'.

The child who limps can have different leg lengths due to overgrowth of one side of the body. There are rare conditions which cause this. Simple things – a child's shoe being too tight, a splinter or plantar wart – can also cause limps!

Children with cerebral palsy affecting one side of their body with weakness and increased tone will have an asymmetric gait – like a stroke. Late presentation of developmental dysplasia of the hip (congenital hip dislocation) can present with a limp in the child from 1 to 5 years.

Sudden onset limps are usually due to trauma, infection of the hip (septic arthritis) or surrounding bone (osteomyelitis). Septic arthritis is a serious condition which needs orthopaedic management and hospitalisation.

Most acute limps are due to a condition called irritable hip, a self-limiting hip condition seen in children of all ages. The findings of unexplained traumatic hip or leg injury in the 1- to 3-year-old child raises concerns of physical child abuse.

An acute painful limp can be caused by leukaemia and will present in the ambulant child more commonly from the age of 5 years onwards. The child will usually be pale, irritable and may have spontaneous bruising.

Chronic hip problems are seen in childhood forms of arthritis. A vascular form of hip problem called Legg–Calve–Perthes disease occurs in older children between 5 and 12 years. The condition of slipped femoral capital epiphysis, where the top of the femur 'falls off', is seen in the adolescent age group from 13 to 19 years.

The 'clumsy' child

Most children when they start to walk spend more time on their bottoms than their legs. They bump into things, trip, stumble and fall. Early childhood is a time when 'clumsiness' is normal.

Children with double-jointedness may have skin and joint laxity. This can be due to a benign form of hypermobility. Ehlers–Danlos syndrome is a rare group of connective tissue disorders with a genetic predisposition. It can present with hypermobility, skin laxity, translucent skin, poor wound healing and joint dislocations. Uncommonly, the heart vessels can be affected. These children can have a 'clumsy' gait and fatigue easily.

The child with fine and gross motor coordination problems can meet the diagnostic criteria for a motor dyspraxia or developmental coordination disorder (DCD). Gait anomalies are common. These children can present with 'clumsy' walks.

Middle ear infections causing a build-up of fluid in the middle ear space can cause balance problems. These are managed by the insertion of grommets, as discussed earlier.

If your child keeps bumping into objects, can they see?

A young girl had a significant vision impairment detected by a paediatric ophthalmologist (eye specialist). Her parents had been concerned that she was poorly coordinated but hadn't detected that she had vision problems. Once ambulant she was very adept at navigating her way around the house by running her hand along the walls of a room. Children are incredibly resilient at accommodating their disabilities.

Bow legs and knock-knees

A child's legs aren't always straight. Your newborn baby's legs will appear 'wonky', but straighten out as they grow. Most children from 1 to 3 years will have some degree of bowing of their lower legs. This is normal.

Bow legs (genu varum), due to a problem with vitamin D or calcium levels, causes rickets. It is rare in Australia.

In knock-knee (genu valgum) deformity, the knees come together and the lower legs stand apart. This is seen commonly in children from 3 to 5 years and usually corrects spontaneously. Severe knock-knee deformity which persists after the age of 10 merits an orthopaedic opinion.

Banana feet (metatarsus adductus)

Curved feet are often seen in infants and children under the age of 2 years. They are the most common form of pigeon toe. This makes children walk with an in-toeing gait. As long as the curve on the foot is flexible and easily correctable, this minor anomaly will self-correct. When we were students, orthopaedic surgeons would just tell parents to put their child's right shoe on the left foot and the left shoe on their right.

In-toeing also occurs when the hips turn in. This is described as inset hips. This developmental condition improves as children grow. You recognise these kids by the way they sit. Their legs are out in front of them with knees bent back in a 'W' shape when they sit down on the floor.

'It's a bird...It's a plane...It's Superman'

Fine motor skills

Children point up in the sky with their index finger to birds, planes, balloons or anything else that they see. This is a defining fine motor milestone called protodeclarative pointing. Its emergence from 12 months signifies good vision, communication and cognitive processing. Children with autism don't always have this milestone, or it is delayed.

This clinical sign is often accompanied by the presence of a precise pincer grip. This allows a child to pick up a small object such as a sultana between the thumb and tip of the index finger. It gives humans an evolutionary advantage over other animals.

To develop good fine motor skills, babies spend a lot of time watching and planning. They need to be able to track the movement of a swinging or mobile object with their eyes before they learn how to grab it. I can recall my own babies lying under their play gym on the mat with *Sesame Street* characters eluding them. The first time they 'whacked' Big Bird I was very excited!

Infants

By 5 to 6 months, babies will reach for an object such as a coloured ring or rattle and grab it. Make sure the rattle is not too top-heavy or it can give your baby a nasty bruise if it hits their head. Babies can hold a rattle but they can't control it. They start to transfer objects from one hand to the other at about 7 months of age.

The 6-month-old baby does lots of banging of objects. When something falls from the highchair, they will follow the movement of the object onto the floor. Tracking fallen objects becomes more accurate from around 9 months. Babies of this age also take a greater interest in people around them. They love throwing things from their highchair tray and enjoy the adults' efforts at picking them up.

Hand dominance

By 13 to 15 months of age, children show a preference for one hand. Most become right-hand dominant. If they develop a very early hand dominance you need to make sure that they are moving both sides of their body well. If a baby has weakness affecting one side of the body (hemiplegia), as you see with a stroke, they develop early hand dominance.

Some forms of cerebral palsy can present like this. A child health nurse, physiotherapist or occupational therapist may pick up on this and refer your child for a medical opinion.

Toddlers

The 15-month-old toddler likes books and pictures and will pat the pages of a favourite picture book. They are keen to hold a pencil or crayon and to make scribbling actions. They enjoy watching and pointing to things.

Scribbling with a pencil becomes more frequent from 18 months. The toddler will sit and 'read' with you, turning several pages of a book at a time. They like to stack two or three blocks into a tower.

At 2 years of age they can stack six or seven small blocks. They can now turn the pages of a book singly and recognise the faces of other people, but not themselves, in photos.

Early childhood

The 3-year-old child is building towers of nine to ten blocks, starting to thread large objects onto string and beginning to cut with toy scissors. A cheap and simple game is to let your 3-year-old put pieces of painted pasta shells onto some thread. They can paint 'abstract' pictures with a large paintbrush. They can copy a circle and draw crude pictures of mum and dad. The towers of blocks now go up to ten or more. It is time for Duplo and Lego!

The pictures of the 4 year old become more refined. When you ask your young child to 'draw a picture of mummy', they will draw a head, body and legs. Arms, fingers and extra details are added. Circles are copied well and your child makes a good attempt at copying a cross. By 5 years squares and crosses are more accurately drawn, and by 6 years a diamond shape.

The 5 year old has become an enthusiastic artist. They will draw and name a number of subjects, usually taken from their external experience. They can colour in neatly between the lines. If a perfectionist, they will destroy inferior works. Children with autism will focus on a theme. Clock faces, numbers, animals, cars, animated or fantasy characters are common.

By 5 to 6 years, children can write several letters and start to write their name. Some letter reversals persist until 6 or 7 years and can be normal. They don't necessarily signify dyslexia.

I find that boys tend to be delayed with their fine motor skills compared with girls. This reflects the busyness of boys and the fussiness of girls. Don't stress if your son is not as good at gluing stickers onto a page as his sister was at the same age.

Don't compare – children are different. They are born with a customised agenda!

Wees and poos

The toileting milestone

The achievement of toileting is the least helpful milestone and not at all predictive of intelligence. Bright kids and those with ADHD often learn to hold on and end up soiling. They are too busy to go to the toilet.

The retention of stool over time can cause the gut to get over-loaded and stretched. The child with chronic constipation soils because they lose the sensation required to empty their bowels, even when they have a distended gut.

Busy, anxious, developmentally delayed and sensory kids will also hold on to their poo or smear it. If your child is sensory and engages in persistent faecal smearing of their cot or room, use other sensory materials to change this pattern of behaviour. Playdough or a squishy toy may divert sensory-seeking behaviours away from their nappy.

Wait until your child is around 3 years before bringing out the playdough if their sensory pattern is to put everything in the mouth. Problematic faecal smearing in a child who has autism or an early global developmental delay (GDD) benefits from intervention with a clinical psychologist or occupational therapist.

To avoid your child being severely constipated, encourage them to eat a varied diet with grains and fruit. This requires you to make healthy food choices for your child. Natural stool softeners, such as benefibre added to cereal or a drink, can help regulate bowel function. Regular toileting helps, especially after meals when the gut is most active.

If constipation is problematic speak further with a child health nurse or your local doctor. Child and parenting support centres and disability services assist. They often run toileting workshops.

Don't force your child to potty-train before they are ready. This can lead to 'potty phobia', toilet avoidance and holding on to stool.

Children around 18 to 24 months start to indicate awareness of bodily functions. Daytime continence precedes night-time continence. Some 'normal' children will continue to have bed-wetting through their early and middle childhood. Most children have dry beds from around 3 to 5 years.

During the day children are dry from around 18 months to 3 years. Some mothers will boast that their child was toilet-trained at 15 to 18 months. I think many of these success stories are due to impeccable toilet timing by the parent. Don't worry if your child is lagging behind.

There is a lot of hype about toilet-training. Most children achieve this milestone when they are developmentally ready.

One evening I tried to put a nappy on my 2-year-old daughter, but she protested, yelling, 'No nappy'. I responded to her kicks by saying,

*'Yes nappy'. I then paused and reflected on my stance. Here was my
child telling me that she didn't need her nappy at night. She was right!*

Some kids are toilet-trained at 2 to 3 years of age and others at
4 to 5 years. It can all be normal.

Wetting issues

The medical term for bedwetting is nocturnal enuresis. It is
common and tends to run in families. Around 20 per cent of
children will wet at age 5 years. But, only about 5 per cent still
wet at 10 years and 1 per cent at 15 years.

If your child is having accidents and wetting their bed at 6 years
of age there are some medical interventions that can help. An
enuresis (bedwetting) alarm can be organised by your child health
nurse, doctor or children's hospital.

If this doesn't work, medications such as Minirin (desmopressin)
can. Discuss these with the child health nurse, family doctor or
paediatrician. Good online parenting resources are available.

Wetting is usually nocturnal and developmental. Bladder,
kidney or spinal cord problems can affect your child's ability to
'hold on'. Constant dribbling of urine or diurnal wetting, where
your child wets in the day and night, needs further investigation.
A paediatric urologist or neurologist can sort out these uncommon
conditions.

Early diabetes mellitus (sugar diabetes) and diabetes insipidus
can cause increased wetting. In both these medical conditions
children drink excessive water. Young children, especially 3- to
5-year-old girls, may go through a stage of compulsive water
drinking. They start to wee more.

Constipation can also affect the ability of the bladder to empty properly. It can predispose your child to develop a urinary tract infection. This can present in the young child as a lapse of bladder training. They start wetting the bed more often.

If your child has been dry at night for a long period and then recommences wetting, you need to consider stressors such as an underlying medical condition, anxiety or even the possibility of developmental trauma, including sexual assault. There will usually be a history suggestive of this, but not always.

Teeth

Little bites

Baby teeth appear around 6 months of age. By 9 months of age many babies have four upper and four lower teeth. This can be variable. The eruption of these teeth can unsettle your baby but shouldn't cause a high temperature. Fevers need to be checked out by a doctor.

Permanent or adult teeth arrive from about 6 to 12 years and wisdom teeth much later, after 16 years of age.

Permanent teeth are important for speech, chewing and good jaw posture and growth. They need to be looked after. This means regular cleaning with a fluoride-based toothpaste, flossing, healthy diets and dental checks. A low-fluoride toothpaste is best prior to the age of 6 years, as children tend to eat the toothpaste when very young.

Children under the age of 2 years need their teeth wiped with some clean gauze to remove food residue. Gently 'brush' the gums and tongue. Start oral hygiene routines early, encouraging your child to use a soft toothbrush for cleaning teeth twice a day.

Some babies will only settle with a dummy (soother or pacifier). Try to wean them from this dependency by 2 to 3 years of age. Never put honey or a sweetener on them. In rare cases raw honey causes infant botulism, a severe bacterial infection caused by *Clostridium botulinum*, which weakens muscles. This is a risk particularly for children under 12 months of age. Dental decay is another potential problem.

Similarly, don't send your child to sleep with a bottle of milk. This can cause midline dental caries. Milk contains 'sugars' which can affect the teeth with prolonged contact. It is best for children to have water if they are thirsty once teeth are cleaned for the night.

Thumb sucking, if persistent, can affect the formation of permanent teeth from the age of 6 years by pushing a tooth out of its correct alignment. It helps to address this habit early.

Doctors aren't taught much about teeth and frequently forget to look at them. Yet teeth can be a source of infection which, if missed, can be problematic in the child with a significant heart murmur, braces or poor immunity. Parents have to care for their child's teeth and ensure regular dental checks are done from an early age.

Children with sensory needs, such as autism, intellectual disability or anxiety, can be distressed by any attempts to clean their teeth. Dental hygiene can be challenging and requires much patience. Some dentists use trained dogs for children to hold while dental work is done. This helps very anxious children relax.

Further information is available from the Australian Dental Association website, the National Maternal and Child Oral Health Resource Center and the American Academy of Pediatric Dentistry. The Speech Therapy Resource – My Child Without Limits website has a section on dental care for babies and young children.

The booklet *Paediatric Dentistry – Dental Care for Children: a Guide for Parents* by Richard Widmer and Gerald Wright is available from The Children's Hospital at Westmead in Sydney. It can also be sourced from the International Association of Paediatric Dentistry website.

Babies aren't born perfect

Looking at life askew

Position your baby's head in different positions for sleep. The baby who always sleeps looking up at the ceiling can end up with a 'flat' head.

Some babies are born with a 'wryneck' due to a preference to turn their head to a particular side. This is described as torticollis. It can occur if your baby is cramped in your uterus because of their size or there is insufficient amniotic fluid (your 'waters').

If your baby always turns their head to one side, ask a child health nurse or doctor to check their neck posture. Muscle-stretching exercises done by you or the physiotherapist gets their neck supple and mobile. If a torticollis is severe the baby develops a tight and shortened muscle on one side of the neck. With time this can affect the facial and skull growth of a baby. They can develop flattening on one side of their head called plagiocephaly. This gives them an egg-shaped head. This is a common and minor problem. It doesn't affect your baby's brain.

Mostly these head changes are subtle. You just turn your baby's head to alternate sides when your baby first goes to sleep. The head remoulds with time, sometimes over a couple of years. Rarely, a moulding helmet is used to get the head 'back into shape'.

If your baby has an odd-shaped head, it is best to ask a health professional for an opinion. Head shapes can be 'normally abnormal', like plagiocephaly, or 'abnormally abnormal' due to an uncommon condition called craniostenosis. This is when the joints between the plates of developing bones in your baby's head stick together too early. This affects the bony growth of the skull. A surgical operation with a specialist who is a craniofacial surgeon may be needed. This is uncommon.

Persistent torticollis can result in facial asymmetry called facial hemihypoplasia. One side of the face can be smaller compared with the other side. One eye can be smaller. It is best to first treat this condition aggressively with physiotherapy. Severe torticollis requires an operation.

Other baby stuff

If you are a worrier, skip this bit. If you read it, maintain perspective. Most babies are born entirely normal.

Baby stuff that worries parents is mostly picked up at the time your newborn baby is examined. But, small things can get missed. If this happens to you, don't be afraid to ask your doctor to take another look. It's a bit like spot-the-difference puzzles. Sometimes the answer is obvious, but you don't always see it, even when you are looking.

Baby poo

Make sure your baby has a bottom hole (anus). If your baby poos, it has one of these. The first few poos look dark green to black in colour and are extremely sticky. This is called meconium. If passed in the amniotic fluid (birth waters) before birth, your baby can become sick, especially if they gasp a mouthful of meconium into their lungs at the time of delivery. This causes breathing problems in the first few days of life. Treatment includes oxygen and antibiotics. Other babies are delivered covered in meconium and are quite content. A paediatrician is asked to assist at the delivery of a baby who has passed meconium during labour.

Meconium passed after birth is a good sign. If a baby doesn't pass meconium within the first forty-eight hours of birth, doctors will check for a thyroid problem or cystic fibrosis. CF is a chronic condition affecting the lungs and digestive system (gut).

Your baby could also be normal! Let the paediatrician do the worrying for you. Just enjoy your baby.

Breathing problems

When a baby struggles to breathe it grunts or breathes very rapidly. This is one of the most common baby problems following delivery. Respiratory distress is caused by infection, prematurity and when meconium is inhaled – called meconium aspiration.

Babies breathe fast, up to sixty times a minute. You and I breathe around twelve to fifteen times a minute. When babies breathe more than eighty times a minute they get tired. They can stop breathing or turn blue or pale.

Premature babies have insufficient surfactant, a lung lubricant produced as babies approach term. It helps the lungs expand. Without it the lungs remain stiff and hard to inflate, a condition called hyaline membrane disease (HMD). If your baby has HMD it will need oxygen and assistance to breathe. A small airway or endotracheal tube is placed in their windpipe and attached to a ventilator. This medical device delivers a specified number of breaths each minute to your baby, the same as when you have an anaesthetic.

Heart problems

Babies can breathe too fast when they have a heart problem. Feeding is difficult. They look pale, mottled in colour or blue (cyanosed). Your baby may have a heart murmur. The pulses in their legs, called the femoral pulses, may be very weak and difficult to feel in the heart condition called coarctation of the aorta. This is caused by an abnormal narrowing of the aorta (the main blood vessel in the body).

About 4 in 10,000 babies are born with this condition. It makes up 4 to 6 per cent of all congenital heart disease and mostly presents from 10 days to 10 weeks of life. Early surgery, before a baby becomes very ill, treats this condition successfully.

Heart murmurs and cardiac conditions are sorted out by your paediatrician and if clinically indicated, by a paediatric cardiologist (heart doctor).

Heart murmurs during early childhood are common. Many disappear with time. Most don't need surgical intervention. Serious heart conditions can be detected on an antenatal ultrasound prior to delivery.

Significant cardiac problems make your baby very sick at 24 or 48 hours of age. They require care in a neonatal intensive care unit.

Fingers and toes

Count how many fingers and toes your baby has. Some babies have an extra toe or thumb. Plastic surgeons have the skills to expertly deal with these small problems. Toes can also be joined together. This can be by partial skin attachment which gives the toes a bifid appearance or webbed look. This does not affect function and is often a familial trait so generally you can ignore it.

Extra things

Some babies have an extra nipple or nipples. A tooth in a newborn baby appears like a small pearly spot or as a red, fleshy lump in the gum.

Small pits or openings in front of your baby's ear or at the base of their spine can be missed. This happens when your baby is still covered with thick vernix, the creamy protective material that protects your baby from its watery environment inside your uterus. Ear pits are only a problem if they get infected, which is rare. We leave them alone.

Sacral pits at the bottom of the spine are only serious if they communicate with the underlying spinal canal and spinal fluid. An ultrasound over the lower part of your baby's spine checks this out.

Skin tags are small pieces of redundant skin often seen around the ears. If large, they are surgically removed. Small ones can be tied off at their base with a piece of suture material and will fall off – like sheep tails.

Eyes

Newborn babies scrunch up their eyes and so they are hard to examine properly. Some babies have a keyhole or tear-drop shaped pupil (the black central hole of the eye). This variant, called a coloboma, is due to a gap or defect in part of the eye structure. It is often benign and affects only a small part of the iris (coloured part of eye). You should still have this checked by an ophthalmologist (eye doctor).

Belly buttons

Your baby may have a small bulge around its belly button (umbilicus). The umbilical cord contains the blood vessels which provide nutrition to a baby during pregnancy. After birth the residual cord forms the umbilicus.

At the six-week check some babies have a moist, sticky area of vascular tissue over their belly button called an umbilical granuloma. This can heal by itself. A small amount of liquid betadine applied to it will hasten the drying process. If larger, an application of silver nitrate can be used. Surgical treatment is uncommon.

If there is a lot of fluid coming from this area of granulating tissue an ultrasound is done to make sure there is no communication of the umbilical stump internally with the bladder.

Boy bits

Male babies are often born with huge-appearing testicles. The scrotal sac is full of fluid, which quickly dissipates. A hydrocoele results when some residual fluid remains around the testicle. Mostly these resolve in the first year of life.

Hypospadias occurs when the urethra, the duct which carries urine from the bladder, falls short of the tip of the penis. Chordee can be associated with this condition and causes the penis to be bent in shape. Hypospadias is a common condition, affecting around 1 in 350 males. No urgent intervention is needed as long as the urine stream is normal and the testes present. A medical opinion is sought to see if future surgical correction is needed.

When the testes are undescended and the hypospadias is severe, the gender of the baby can be uncertain. This is clearly a sensitive time for parents. Expert specialist opinion is a priority. This is provided by a paediatric endocrinologist and surgeon.

Skin

In the first few days to 2 weeks after birth some babies develop a rash called toxic erythema of the newborn. This is benign and self-resolving. It starts on the face and extends to the trunk and limbs but usually spares the palms of the hands and soles of the feet. The rash consists of a combination of flat red patches, small red bumps and pustules.

Staphylococcal scalded skin syndrome is a serious skin rash which can occur in newborns, infants and young children. An affected baby will have a red rash with pustules that blister. They will have a high temperature and be irritable. Management involves hospitalisation and antibiotics.

Pustules in the newborn baby which enlarge quickly can be caused by a *Streptococcus* or *Staphylococcus* bacterial skin infection. Early treatment is with topical Betadine, an antiseptic, if lesions are small, or an oral antibiotic if lesions are spreading. More aggressive antibiotic treatment will be needed if your baby becomes unwell.

A localised area of skin deficit on your baby's scalp is known as aplasia cutis congenital. This is rare. The underlying bony skull can be involved. These skin lesions appear like punched-out areas. They are usually small and heal by scarring. If large, a surgical opinion is sought.

Harlequin phenomenon is uncommon and seen mostly in newborn babies. The skin colour will suddenly change in a specific or large part of the baby's body. Classically, this occurs down the midline of the body dividing your baby's skin into two different colours. It is transient and doesn't harm your baby.

Harlequin ichthyosis is a rare skin condition characterised by the baby having very thickened and altered skin.

Strawberry naevi or haemangiomas are raised red skin lesions consisting of lots of small blood vessels. They look like strawberries, hence their name. They are common and appear from one to four weeks after birth on the head, neck and other areas. They grow for weeks or months and then start to involute and disappear. As they shrink pale areas appear in them. This occurs during the first and sometimes second year of life. Rarely, these spots enlarge rapidly and need dermatological or surgical intervention. These skin lesions often have a bluish component. You can feel them under the skin.

Big heads

If your baby's head looks big it probably is, in the same way that some heads look small. Before panicking, look around the family table and see if anyone else has a big head. They probably do. Most often this is a familial trait.

Hydrocephalus

Big heads are not always normal. Rapid head growth is seen in the uncommon condition hydrocephalus. Colloquially, this is known as 'water on the brain' and is due to an increase in brain fluid. Your baby's skull is made up of soft plates of bones which haven't yet joined solidly together. They can move and expand if the brain is under pressure.

In hydrocephalus, prominent veins appear on a baby's head and the 'soft spot' (anterior fontanelle) becomes tense. Severe brain pressure creates the clinical sign of 'sun-setting' eyes. The whites of the baby's eyes become very prominent. The coloured part or iris sits low in the eye sockets. The baby with these rare signs is very ill and presents with an irritable cry, vomiting and drowsiness. They can have a seizure (fit).

Genetic disorders

Genetic conditions with large heads such as Sotos syndrome or Dandy–Walker malformation, a condition with large brain cysts, are rare. Before you do an internet search for these diagnoses, take a breath and look at your baby. If they are reaching expected milestones – feeding, looking and babbling – they are most likely normal.

Low tone

Big heads can make it harder for your baby to sit up. They might have head lag and be slower to reach their gross motor milestones. Their head will flop back when you pull them up from a flat surface. This also happens when babies are floppy due to low tone. They will sit, crawl and walk later.

Uncommon medical conditions which present with low tone include specific types of cerebral palsy, rare metabolic and storage disorders, hypothyroidism (low thyroid function), and, as previously discussed, SMA and Duchenne muscular dystrophy.

Baby checks

Newborn examination and infant healthcare is done by a midwife, infant health nurse, GP, paediatrician or hospital training doctor. This duty must be performed with care, discretion, confidence, honesty and consistency. Not all doctors will be able to pick up what is wrong with your baby. You may have to ask for a second opinion.

Sometimes the doctor caring for your baby will consult another doctor. This doesn't mean they're a bad doctor. It means that they recognise their limitations and are not too proud to ask for advice or support.

Too much information can be detrimental to the emotional health of a young mother. Mothers who develop postnatal depression can present as very anxious about the health and wellbeing of their baby. Doctors and child health nurses must not fuel this anxiety.

The role of the child health nurse in monitoring your child's early development is important. They are trained to pick up what is normal and what is not normal. Your job is to nurture and enjoy your baby.

Childhood ills and spills

Sick children

Children are at risk from infection and accidental trauma in the first five years of childhood. Some children are the victims of non-accidental trauma due to family violence. Don't read about the potential disasters of childhood if you have just had a baby. A child's early years are mostly spent being happy and healthy.

Most childhood deaths occur in infants less than 12 months and are related to factors occurring before, during or at birth, or genetic abnormalities that result in congenital defects. These are abnormalities seen in newborn babies. They include abnormal chromosomal combinations not compatible with life. Infancy is a time when parents worry about SIDS.

Once your baby has safely reached 12 months they have an excellent chance of a healthy life. Australia provides quality healthcare for mothers and babies, a fact not always acknowledged.

Unexpected risks for children include motor vehicle accidents, drownings and assaults due to non-accidental injury and poisoning.

Childhood cancer rates are a significant cause of childhood death. Burns and falls can be problematic.

Parents can't completely childproof their homes, but they can make them considerably safer by spending some time and thought on childhood hazards. Safety precautions include securing lithium button batteries in remote controls. These can be deadly if swallowed. Discarded cigarette butts, prescribed medications, washing powders, bleach, toilet cleaner and alcohol are also toxic to children.

I have listed a number of potential and largely preventable childhood dangers at the end of this section.

Significant childhood infections

Severe bacterial infection can make children extremely ill and on occasion, even when treated, can result in disability and death. It is important to detect these illnesses early. This means listening and acting when a parent is concerned about their child.

Virulent bacteria include *Neisseria meningitidis,* the pathogen in life-threatening meningococcal disease, *Streptococcus pneumoniae, Staphylococcus aureus* and *Haemophilus influenzae.* Group B streptococcal infection continues to be a threat to newborn babies. All these bacteria can cause meningitis.

The symptoms of meningitis are fever, vomiting, headache, photophobia (light sensitivity) and a stiff neck. Affected children look sick and get sicker rapidly. Very young children don't always have the sign of a stiff neck, so detecting meningitis in them is harder.

A rash can be present in meningococcal meningitis. It is a distinctive pinpoint red or rapidly evolving purple rash that does not blanch and often first appears in hands, feet and limbs.

Sometimes there is no rash. A child is just pale and very ill. Meningococcal disease is a medical emergency. If you suspect this take your child to the closest doctor or emergency department. Don't waste valuable time trying to contact a helpline.

The good news is that your baby has an immune system and your antibodies help protect them in the early weeks of life. Severe bacterial infections need urgent antibiotic treatment. We also live in a country with excellent healthcare, diligent immunisation programs and competent health professionals.

Is your baby too hot?

Babies in the first few weeks of life with a temperature should be assessed by a doctor. They could have a urinary tract infection or blood infection (sepsis). High temperatures, especially those over 38 °C, can't be dismissed as a viral infection until blood tests and urine tests are done. Some babies need to have a lumbar puncture (spinal tap) to exclude meningitis.

The sick baby is quiet, feeds poorly, vomits, look pale or mottled in colour and has a high temperature. Very ill babies can have low temperatures of 35 °C and a rapid and irregular breathing rate. They have lots of watery stools or fewer wet and dirty nappies, especially if they are vomiting frequently. A change in your baby's behaviour will indicate that your baby is not well.

The baby who vomits blood or green bile and the young child who passes a sticky, bloodied stool and is unwell has to be seen by a doctor. These clinical signs could indicate a serious surgical condition such as intussusception (twist in the gut) or pyloric stenosis (stomach outlet blockage). Babies with an intussusception look pale and can deteriorate extremely quickly. They require urgent radiological and surgical intervention.

Babies and premature babies who have a fever during the first six weeks need the expertise of an experienced doctor or paediatrician. If you are worried about your infant, attend the emergency department of your nearest hospital, preferably a children's hospital.

Remote medicine

Families living outside metropolitan areas can feel scared and isolated when sickness strikes. In remote parts of Australia these families have the resources of regional nursing posts, rural hospitals and the Royal Flying Doctor Service.

Telemedicine and Skype deliver medical advice and limited assessment to people living in country towns and outback places. These are great innovations but can never replace the benefits of face-to-face medical consultation.

Immunisation

Childhood immunisation prevents children from contracting disabling diseases such as polio, epiglottitis, measles, mumps, rubella, chicken pox, pertussis (whooping cough), diphtheria, tetanus and some forms of meningitis.

Epiglottitis, a life-threatening upper-airway disease, is now rare because of vaccination and won't have been seen by newly graduated doctors. Polio has nearly been eradicated and smallpox officially has.

Mumps is an infectious disease that affects the parotid glands. They produce saliva, which helps break food down. Mumps makes eating painful and causes very high temperatures. In males it can result in painful testicles and infertility. It can also cause hearing loss. A vaccination became available for mumps in Australia in 1981.

Polio vaccines became available in 1956, the same year of Australia's last polio epidemic.

When I was a medical student I met a woman who had contracted polio, an infection caused by a virus called an enterovirus. Polio can cause minimal symptoms, meningitis or paralysis of single muscle groups. In this woman it had affected her respiratory muscles. She was unable to breathe by herself and was confined to an 'iron lung', a non-invasive form of mechanical ventilation. It consisted of a circumferential chamber in which a patient lay enclosed with only their head and neck exposed.

This woman resided as a permanent patient at the now-closed Fairfield Infectious Diseases Hospital in Melbourne.

Her plight from a 'simple' preventable infection left an indelible memory.

People who choose not to vaccinate their children against childhood infectious diseases have been protected by good herd or general immunity within the community.

Global vaccination has eradicated the disfiguring disease of smallpox and nearly eradicated polio. But in 2013 and 2014, polio has started to bounce back in some countries, including in Asia, Africa and the Middle East. With international travel, it is possible that your non-immunised child or teenager could be exposed to it. You need to be aware of this. Measles has also become more common in non-vaccinated travellers.

Household threats

Houses are not fail-safe places for children. Typical household hazards can be as simple as a large laundry bucket which has sufficient stability for a toddler to tumble into headfirst. They can potentially drown in a few centimetres of water. The toddler doesn't have the body mass or strength to get out of a large bucket unassisted.

Other dangers include free-hanging cords from blinds and curtains in which children can become entangled. Parents need to keep these cords well secured.

Button batteries, such as those in remote controls, are diabolically dangerous. They can corrode through the lining of a child's oesophagus or stomach. They have resulted in the deaths of young children under the age of 5 years.

If you suspect a child has swallowed one of these batteries, it is a medical emergency. Go straight to the nearest hospital and get immediate help. I will list other common hazards at the end of this chapter.

Emotional and social milestones

Emotional meltdowns and showdowns

The temper tantrums of the 2 to 3 year old become the 'emotional meltdown' of the 4 to 6 year old. They become the 'acting out' behaviour of the emotionally dysregulated 7 to 12 year old. In adolescence and emerging adulthood, these same emotional crises can be seen in generalised anxiety disorders (GADs), depressive states and disordered eating behaviours. In adult life they tend to be called personality disorders.

The tag of 'naughty' or 'oppositional' is often given to the disruptive and hyperactive child with suspected ADHD, autism or family dysfunction. The early school records of these children are frequently highlighted with red or black notes, requests for early parent–teacher interviews and school suspensions. Some of these children are sent home from kindergarten or pre-primary for biting, hitting or throwing objects at students or teachers.

It is not logical to sort out the problems of the complex, poorly behaved pre-primary-school child by rewarding them with absence from school for biting or spitting. If I were in the shoes of that child I would bite every day so I could be sent home to stay with my mum.

We have all witnessed those awkward parenting moments when we wish we had chosen to walk down a different aisle of the supermarket. Some children don't like shopping. If you can, don't take them with you. Do something that you both enjoy. It will make a happier and more enduring memory. I often hear young children crying out to their parent, 'How much longer? I'm tired, can we go home now?'

Worse is when a tired parent shoves their smartphone in the face of their toddler and keeps them captive, strapped tightly in their stroller. Another opportunity to talk, walk, laugh and communicate with a child has been lost.

It is better to acknowledge defeat, leave the shopping centre and go to a park and play. Return home and make biscuits, muffins or slices rather than buying them. This requires time, planning and patience. Most parents run out of these commodities. I have been at fault of taking the easy route by dropping in on a fast-food outlet. Yet, it wouldn't have taken long to make a toasted sandwich, boil an egg or put together a salad at home.

Listen to small voices

Listen to your child even before they learn to talk. Never underestimate the ability of an infant to learn from observation. The developing brain of a young child has the potential to become the future inventor, innovator, mathematician, musician, actor, designer, creator or carer. Babies are born with the ability to learn holistically. They utilise all their senses to integrate their world of noises, images and emotions. Babies learn through what they see, hear, touch, taste, smell and feel.

Alzheimer's Australia Western Australian Chief Executive Rhonda Parker was quoted as saying, 'It is true that someone with dementia may not be able to remember what you said. But they'll always remember how you make them feel'. Babies also pick up the emotional vibes of those around them. Babies can respond to the way we interact with them even before they are born.

I remember one night watching the film The Terminator *starring Arnold Schwarzenegger. I was in the last thirteen weeks of my pregnancy. There was a film sequence of noise and violence. My unborn child woke up, kicked and somersaulted. I was glad that she could hear, but I wondered whether she was scared. You might prefer to let your baby listen to Mozart and Bach!*

Teach your child to listen

Never underestimate the ability of the young child to listen, learn and remember. You won't always be there to protect them, so give them life skills early.

When I was working in private general practice in Melbourne in 1986, I received a phone call at the medical centre early one morning. A 4-year-old boy told me that he couldn't rouse his mother. She had diabetes and had told him how to contact our surgery if she was ill.

He was able to give his home address. I turned up in unison with the ambulance. She had a very low blood sugar and responded when I gave her some intravenous dextrose (sugar). This young boy had listened to his mother's instructions. He saved his mother's life.

Children can also be good teachers. They listen and absorb words, feelings and the actions around them. It is important that as adults we are on our best behaviour in front of impressionable children.

I saw a young child stand up to a very tall and intimidating orthopaedic surgeon. He was gruff and prickly on the outside but as malleable as a marshmallow beneath his skin. He often threw a few expletives around. I recall 'bloody' was his favourite this particular day.

After hurling a couple of these expletives, the 5 year old stood up to her full tiny height, glared at him and made the simple statement: 'Choose another word'.

There was a moment of silence and reflection, abruptly broken by the chortles from the grandfather. She had a win and a convert that day.

Burnt toast, cold coffee and silent pauses

Beware the sound of silence

The years from 0 to 5 are permeated by the lingering waft of burnt toast and the metallic taste of cold coffee. This is when a mother, father or carer must remain hypervigilant and fight fatigue, especially when caring for the busy or inquisitive child.

Every parent will tell you to beware the 'sound of silence' in the 2- to 4-year-old child.

A colleague still reflects on her decision to return home after leaving for work. Her husband was in charge of their young daughter. Upon her

return, the house was silent. In that defining moment they raced out to
the backyard pool. The pool gate was swinging and their daughter was
floating quietly in the water, about to drown.

Parental intuition is a precious gift. We should learn to
acknowledge it without allowing our own anxieties to distort its
value. It saved one child that day.

Parental responsibility is as much about vigilance as love and
nurture. When a parent's awareness is blunted by alcohol, drugs,
fatigue, anxiety and depression, a child's safety is compromised.

School readiness

Cognition and learning

Schools expect parents to teach their children the cognitive, social
and emotional skills that prepare them for learning. Children need
to be able to listen, follow simple instructions, play, share and
socialise. School-age children require good adaptive skills to make
them independent for toileting and eating.

If parents fail to do this, their child is socially, emotionally and
academically behind upon school entry.

Part of this pre-school preparation involves parents reading
alongside their children, singing nursery rhymes, playing card
games and encouraging creative make-believe play. It is important to provide a rich pre-literacy environment within our homes.
This is not happening enough. Studies have shown that children
in their second year of life in a literacy-poor environment have
an increased risk of reading problems including reading comprehension in later childhood.

Favourite books

My kids liked the rhyming story *A Sausage Went for a Walk* written by Ellisha Majid and illustrated by Peter Kendall. By popular request we wore out the *Slinky Malinki* books by Lynley Dodd and books by Mem Fox such as *Shoes from Grandpa* and *Tough Boris.*

I liked the story about Boris, a scary pirate who is not afraid to cry, because the child who meets Boris is not afraid to cry either. What a great message for kids about emotional resilience.

Pamela Allen's *Who Sank the Boat* and *The Very Hungry Caterpillar* by Eric Carle are classic children's reads. It is sad that some nursery schools in the United Kingdom have shunned the 'hungry caterpillar' because he is too greedy and could make children over-eat and become obese!

Anticipatory books, such as the lift-the-flap book *Hide and Seek* by Jez Alborough and *Spot Bakes a Cake* by Eric Hill, are good for kids, especially around 12 to 18 months when they are developing memory.

Sequencing stories, such as *Goldilocks and the Three Bears* and *We're Going on a Bear Hunt* by Michael Rosen and Helen Oxenbury, are important for the development of language. They are useful narratives for kindy, pre-primary and year 1 students. They are also good for babies!

Many of these books have a rhythmical beat which assists a child to retain phrases in their phonetic memory. That is why the Dr Seuss series of books have remained so popular. They inspire a child's imagination with timeless characters that make phonics, rhyme and reading fun.

The key to getting a child to read is to read with them. Show your child that you like reading as well. Ensure they have access to electronic and paper books.

The brightness of electronic screens can potentially affect the sleep cycle of a young child, so I prefer night-time stories to be from paper books. All children benefit from the tactile experience of a book. They enjoy seeing the words in front of them disappear as they turn each page and new ones appear.

Social stories

Books provide children with social stories – visual pictures that tell kids what to do. They spark imagination and foster the love of reading. Make sure that you prioritise this early learning experience for your child.

Children don't learn to read by osmosis or by watching an electronic screen which does their thinking for them. This is 'lazy learning'. Reading and early learning apps supplement the hard slog of physical reading but lack the social tips gained by reading with a parent.

A child and their parent need to sit and enjoy at least 10 minutes of 'alongside reading' each day. This provides time for a child to hear sounds and words and to work out how they go together to make meaningful sentences. It allows a child to ask questions, think and dream. It provides a safe environment for the teaching of 'social stories'.

Books such as *Don't Think About Purple Elephants* by Susan Whelan, *When Sophie Gets Angry* by Molly Bang and the series of Jack books on bullying by Susanne Gervay, including *I Am Jack*, are 'social stories' for children. They provide strategies and a safety net to address their fears and anxieties.

Award-winning Western Australian children's author and educator Jan Ramage has written a number of books that incite a social conscience in children. They include the books, *Deepsea Whale Rescue* and *Tuart Dwellers*.

I have listed other book suggestions in the bibliography section.

Education – an external developmental influence

Age criteria for school entry vary slightly between states and territories. Generally, children of 3 to 4 years can enter a kindergarten program and a child of 5 years can start a preparatory or pre-primary year. Primary school starts the year your child turns 6 and extends from year 1 to year 6. Secondary school is from year 7 to year 12. Students commence high school at 12 years of age and complete school at 18.

Most families choose a structured classroom-learning format for their child upon compulsory school entry. You will need to make choices about early-learning programs before your child turns 3. These include formal day-care placements and private pre-kindergartens.

There is increased early emphasis on the development of numeracy and literacy with standardised testing of these core-learning areas on entry to formal schooling in pre-primary. Children are forced to read during their pre-primary school year, even if they don't have the pre-literacy skills to do this. These children become highly anxious and are set up to fail.

Some families choose schools which adopt a greater emphasis on play in the early childhood curriculum, in either the public or private school system. Other families need access to education support facilities or specialised funded autism units if their child has a significant physical or intellectual disability.

Language centres

Language development centres provide targeted and intensive intervention for students with isolated language delay not due to autism. Students have normal intelligence. Applications are made by a speech pathologist with support from a clinical psychologist or paediatrician.

Alternative education options

Montessori schools assist children to learn by allowing them to follow their own natural curiosity, watch and listen to older children and not to be forced to learn before they are psychologically ready. They want children to love learning.

The Reggio Emilia philosophy embraces the relationship between the child, their family and learning.

Steiner schools focus on engaging students by teaching methods through the arts such as music, movement, drama, speech and poetry.

Home schooling

Home schooling is often chosen by families on religious grounds, for philosophical reasons or because their child has autism. It can be a lifeline for families in transition between schools.

Increasingly, families who have a child failing in the conventional school system because of bullying, anxiety or learning problems view home-based education as an opportunity to teach their primary school child how to read, write and compute in a 'safe' environment. Many of these children re-enter mainstream schooling. Those too traumatised by work or social anxiety can't.

Mainstream schooling

Most children go to their local public school, particularly during the primary years. Gifted and talented education schools are government schools that specialise in academic excellence, visual arts, music, drama, computer science and sport. Entry is by successful application based on academic assessment and audition.

There are also a large number of children who attend private Catholic and non-Catholic private schools.

School choice

All these education opportunities have their merits. Parents decide which school is the best fit for their child. It should not be about which school sits highest on league tables. School choice is best made on emotional and social grounds.

There are practical considerations. With traffic increasing exponentially, why would you drive your primary school child away from their potential peer group to a school remote from where you live? This may be necessary in high school to accommodate your teenage child's needs. Think carefully about doing this in the early years.

Music – a lifelong influence

Music offers a channel for children to connect to their innate feelings and create their unique voice. This assists them in finding a place in the world. There are gifted and innovative early childhood music teachers in Australia. They conduct music classes for children from birth to 5 years. Many of these programs are based on the philosophies of Émile Jaques-Dalcroze, Zoltán Kodály and Carl Orff. They aspire to help children connect with themselves and others through song, dance, movement and play.

Website addresses of innovative music classes are provided in the resource section of this book.

Maternal dilemmas

Parental disempowerment

Work commitments necessitate outsourcing of parental care and responsibility. This can be an agonising decision for any parent. There is no place for judgement when a parent returns to work and has to arrange childcare placements.

Some people presume that a mother's priority is to give up work and care exclusively for her child. This is not always possible or even in the best interests of some women. There needs to be a balance and preparedness for compromise. Many families share parenting responsibility and accept fewer paid work hours.

It is important to consider how a child will change your relationship with your partner, family, friends, career and yourself. You need to plan how to accommodate the needs of a child and maintain the integrity of your relationships.

Many grandparents find themselves caught up in the expectations of shared child rearing. Some grandparents feel displaced and even ostracised by their own children and step-children. The experience of their parenting is belittled and even resented. They face the delicate balance of stepping back to allow their children to parent but jumping in when needed. There is a major shift in loyalty within some families. A breakdown of communication and connectivity can occur. This cannot always be rectified.

Never take family for granted. Family relationship is trans-generational and ongoing. Consistent 'parenting' when raising a child is vital, especially when extended family share this role and where there is parental separation. This is achievable with careful planning and by maintaining a stance of childhood advocacy above parental self-interest.

When parents separate it is very important that children know the new rules as quickly as possible. Parents will have different parenting styles, but the fundamental rules must be retained. They include kindness, consistency, firm but fair boundaries, positive and reflective parenting, routine without rigidity and minimal choices.

This is not always possible, particularly in the setting of acrimonious parental separation. The result is child and adult anxiety, conflict within households, sibling rivalry and family dysfunction.

You need your family when you raise children. The responsibility of parenthood doesn't cease when a child finishes school. Sometimes it can be even more challenging and demanding when the emerging young adult faces a battle with emotional, social or physical turmoil.

Work choices and hard choices for mothers

Some professional women have already spent a significant time investment in their career when they have a child.

The self-identity and social confidence of women in high-achieving professional roles can be based on professional success. Some find it daunting to mingle with other mothers, do canteen rosters, help at toy libraries and join mother groups. They feel displaced and socially awkward with other mothers who organise picnics, car pool, run children's parties, make cupcakes, sew great costumes and do great hair.

The transition period from profession to motherhood requires good friends, supportive family and helpful colleagues. This helps mothers stumble through the difficult early years.

Reflect carefully on childcare arrangements before the birth of your child. It is a painful and difficult decision to trust your baby to the care of another, even if they are family. Be flexible, as plans change if your baby is born prematurely or with a significant illness, disability or congenital defect.

Childcare in homes

Some families employ a nanny or au pair to look after a child within their own home. If you choose this option, be meticulous in screening that person. Check references. Have a formal written contract of employment.

Professional couples are good in their field. They can be naïve and overly trusting when inviting a stranger into their home to care for their child. If you are lucky, your nanny will be the linchpin for your family. You will form an enduring relationship with them. Value and respect a good and reliable carer. Don't be mean with your remuneration, even if this means you see little money left out of your own pay packet. A good carer is the best investment you are likely to make and hard to find.

Extended family members and friends are increasingly called upon to care for children during the early years. They become an integral part of how a family functions. Sadly, 'family' does not always equate with 'safe'. A parent's duty is to ensure their child is safe. That is a priority that must always come above family.

Family day care

Other families prefer the security of many eyes for their child and choose a formal day-care centre or crèche. Don't be complacent in this choice. There have been publicly reported cases of child abuse in registered day-care centres and holiday resorts.

Family day care with a registered carer who looks after a limited number of children within their home appeals to some families. You must still feel comfortable and secure with your choice of carer.

Feeling isolated

It is an onerous task to raise children without backup from the village. Try to network while your child is young. Avoid being self-sufficient. Your partner will want to take off six weeks when you first have a baby, but it might be better for them to take less leave initially and have some in reserve for later. This will give you time to develop your own mothering strategies and cope when your partner returns to work. Mothers suffering with postnatal depression will require intensive early and sustained support from family and health professionals.

Some of my most treasured friendships have been those where my friends have forgotten that I am a paediatrician. They just treat me as a mother and see my needs.

When I left hospital with my first baby I initially felt quite alone. Our extended families were interstate and many of my professional friends were busy working. As a paediatrician I knew a lot about the physical needs of babies but this didn't prepare me for the isolation of having one.

I learned that having a baby places you in a separate social space. When I had to go the shops and park my car, I developed a greater understanding of how it must feel to have a disability. I had to seek ramps and easy-to-park areas. Some retailers viewed babies as a liability. Without the mask of my profession I experienced the put-downs that many mothers experience in the public domain.

At the time, breastfeeding in public was frowned upon. Now, widespread acceptance of breastfeeding is a positive consequence of our social shift.

Social connectivity
What made a difference to me as a naïve mother was the social connectivity from neighbours, the infant health nurse, friends and the kinship from early mothers' groups.

One of my friends, a paediatric intensive care nurse, dropped into my home one day with morning tea. She took charge, as ICU nurses do, and made me a cup of coffee, bathed my baby, changed her nappy and had a chat. It is the little things that can make a difference. Never underestimate the smile, kind words, looks and practical actions that can change a mother's day.

Some mothers choose to remain at home full-time with their child for as long as they can. If you do this, hold off on any major expensive home renovations and prioritise your focus on being at home with your child. A 1-year-old child won't know whether there are rectified tiles in the bathroom, or shadow line cornices. However, they will carry with them a sense of how they felt in their early home environment.

There is a balance between adopting a micromanagement approach to child raising and sound, sensible preparation for parenthood. Take time to rest and ponder in the last few weeks at home before you have your baby. Some women work up until their due date or due to premature labour never get to have the valuable quiet time in preparation for childbirth. Labour is hard and tiring work – physically and emotionally. It helps to be fit and rested before undertaking it.

The vulnerability of childhood

Postnatal depression

Listening to your baby requires you to listen to the silence of your child as closely as you would their cries. The quiet baby who feeds, sleeps and is not demanding may not be the perfect baby. They could have problems with their vision or hearing, or lack the sensory stimulation of conversation, eye contact, play and attention. This can occur when a mother is suffering from postnatal depression. It is seen when a mother is physically and mentally exhausted from sleep deprivation and the demands of caring for a newborn baby.

Postnatal depression can have a significant impact on mothers, babies and families. It is an area of great complexity and beyond the boundaries of this book. There are excellent resources and supports to assist mothers who suffer with depression. Key lifeline people are partners, family, friends, neighbours, child health nurses, midwives, obstetricians, family doctors, psychiatrists, mental health nurses, social workers and psychologists.

Developmental trauma

A family can experience parental separation, domestic violence, financial hardship, physical illness or even death. Whilst physical abuse is overt, emotional neglect and abuse is covert and can be more detrimental to a child's development. Raising a child in any of these adverse circumstances is difficult.

Developmental trauma is increasingly recognised, although not yet clearly defined in the *Diagnostic and Statistical Manual of Mental Disorders, Fifth Edition (DSM-5)* classification of mental disorders. Awareness, prevention and effective management of childhood trauma is a priority. This enables children to develop emotional resilience and become effective young adults.

Greater recognition and specialised training is needed in this area. Paediatricians and child psychiatrists can make a difference to families. Clinical psychologists, families, educators, police and the wider community assist. They connect, help and save children subjected to domestic violence. Professionals provide support and non-judgemental intervention.

The Australian Human Rights Commission recognises the rights of the child to be raised in a safe environment. Refugee status should not exclude a child from this right. It is our moral, ethical and human responsibility to care for our children. Developmental trauma happens within the best and the worst of homes. Social boundaries do not halt its sinister and potentially devastating effect.

Protect childhood

The early childhood years are crucial for the strong emotional, social and physical growth of a child. Positive childhood memories protect children in later life.

Family life is an integral part of the making of a child's memories. Children can store highly emotive visual images forever.

The media has a vital role in conveying this message and ensuring that boys grow up respecting their sisters, mothers and daughters. In a press conference, Prime Minister Malcolm Turnbull made the statement: 'Disrespecting women does not always result in violence against women. But all violence begins with disrespecting women'.

Social media influences how young adults treat one another. Public opinion shouts out against rape culture and the denigration of women. Yet, young adults applaud inferior comedians who chase 'likes' by 'slut-shaming' and use the 'c word' as their artistic signature.

To value children we have to change our behaviours, address mental health issues and work to make cohesive, functional families. Respect needs to be grown at home.

Emotional abuse

It can be very difficult to breach the contours of a tight bubble of privacy around some families, particularly where there is covert emotional abuse. In these situations we need to listen to the children and act on behalf of the child when required.

The concerns of other family members should be heard. Each voice within a family tells a different story.

We must address the consequences of developmental trauma in children, whether this is inflicted in foster placements, refugee camps or 'normal' homes.

Emotional abuse in a young child is often hidden. It occurs when a child from a young age experiences parental anger, inconsistent and cold parental responses and bullying. This can be from parents or siblings. These children become anxious.

We have talked about the language of anxiety in young children. It is expressed with social and emotional withdrawal, fears and irrational worries, paranoia and phobic behaviours or the emergence of controlling and obsessive behaviours.

Self-harm

The anxious, angry or sad child self-harms to release their stress. A young child head bangs, bites or scratches. The older child pinches, cuts and burns.

This pattern of behaviour can escalate and when fuelled by depression can lead to a suicide attempt or successful suicide, even in a young child.

Stable parenting puts in place preventive measures to assist children develop strong emotional resilience to combat self-harm behaviours. External assistance is provided by psychologists and psychiatrists.

Most parents who face a child in 'meltdown' mode struggle to think reflectively. They nag, bellow and shout at their child. This is not their fault. It is a human flaw. No one walks in their shoes. We have to make sure that professional support is available to redirect the energy of parents into optimal ways of helping their children.

Record childhood

When you have children, complete a baby book for each child. When those babies are teenagers they will seek confirmation that you can remember what they were like and the funny things they did as babies.

You think you will never forget what your child did at the various childhood stages, or how much they weighed, but you will.

Don't lie to children

Be honest with your teenage son or daughter. This helps foster trust. In her insightful and timeless book *The Magic Years*, written more than 50 years ago, Selma H. Fraiberg wrote about the importance of telling children the truth, especially when it came to death. If a child's pet died, she advised that the child should be told. She made the powerful statement that 'in our efforts to protect children from painful emotions we may deprive them of their own best means of mastering painful experiences'.

You can't always rescue children from their emotions. Children have to learn how to deal with their feelings, including those relating to death. Tears are a great release for sadness. As adults, we are there to help.

The gift of childhood is fragile

Tragedy afflicts some families during the early childhood years. Risk factors are injury and death through non-accidental and accidental injury, motor vehicle accidents and medical causes such as serious infections.

Sometimes life just takes care of children. Sometimes it doesn't. It's not logical, fair or reasonable. It's just the way it is.

One of our cats used up his nine lives before they were due and passed on the spare ones to the cat who remained behind. Maybe this is what children do too. Some children can be lucky and some aren't. No explanation can dissipate grief when a child dies. It is always horrible.

Growing roots

Family traditions

Develop family traditions, especially if you are socially isolated. This helps establish good communication within families and is protective for children. Traditions can be as simple as making muffins or pancakes on weekend mornings with your children, walking by the water, riding bikes or playing in a park. This enables your family to become familiar with the physical parameters of the neighbourhood and to meet people in the community.

Maintaining a healthy lifestyle means having meals together, a good sleeping pattern and time for exercise and leisure. This helps raise happy children. Play board games on a Friday night such as Scrabble, Dominoes and Rummikub. Try card games such as Uno, Snap, 500, Euchre or Crib.

Some of my favourite childhood memories relate to doing simple things, such as staying at my grandmother's house over the Christmas holidays and listening to the waves crashing down on the sandy beach at the end of her street. Inevitably it is the perception of the child that forms a positive and happy childhood memory. It is not money, having lots of things or expensive holidays. It is silly stuff, trivia and nonsense that kids remember.

Practise effective use of leisure time with your partner so that it is part of your life routine before children. This can be a good strategy when you have a busy partner who never has time, or takes time to relax. If they don't learn to do this before children, you may find yourself being the primary caregiver. This is not conducive to a strong partnership. Women have a lot of power in how they can run the household, but they need to think, plan and develop strategies which will create a healthy child-raising environment.

If you need empowerment, reflect on the character Maria Portokalos in the film *My Big Fat Greek Wedding*. When discussing family hierarchy, she says, 'The man is the head, but the woman is the neck. And, she can turn the head any way she wants'.

Give your children stable roots. Familiarity of home and neighbourhood is comforting for children. It gives them a sense of belonging. Plant a deciduous tree. It will provide shelter and sustenance for the local bird life, bring music into your garden and provide shade and protection for your children. It will deliver privacy from neighbours, a proxy cubby for kids, a scratching pole for your pets and leaves to sweep up when you retire.

DOs – 0 to 5 years

Do

- prepare for parenthood
- plan kid-free time
- recognise the needs of all those within your family but don't forget your own
- lower your expectations when you have a baby
- set achievable parenting goals
- learn the difference between mess and dirt
- wear your breastmilk-stained top as a badge of honour
- remember that babies don't need to be dressed perfectly
- try 'tummy time' at each nappy change
- practise calm, consistent and reflective parenting
- be kind – love and believe in your child
- learn to read the language of your young child by interpreting their behaviours
- walk and run, play, imagine and explore
- turn off the TV and DVD and remove the iPad, computer and tablet
- allow a child to fail so that they learn to succeed
- stamp out narcissism
- write down strategies that work for you and your child in a book for future reference
- keep an affirmation book
- start your own family traditions
- remember that you don't live in a *Vogue* magazine!
- add a pet to your family
- attend to the small things so that the big changes will be possible
- recite 'to do nothing is to gain little'
- borrow the mantra – 'take the pettiness out of littleness and the littleness out of pettiness'

DON'Ts – 0 to 5 years

Don't

- lose the 'to dos' list!
- give up on your child
- be afraid of your toddler
- fret over the small things
- be an overreactive parent
- fuel your child's anxiety with your own
- be a 'fixer' who tries to protect their child from the lessons of life
- nag – listen to your child
- make your child's development a competition
- use shopping trolleys without the use of the provided child restraints
- apologise for breastfeeding your baby
- be afraid to ask for help when you need it
- take your partner or family relationship for granted

Potential childhood risks – 0 to 5 years

Ingestions and inhalations

- button batteries from remote controls contain lithium – caustic if swallowed and can cause death
- medications – paracetamol (Panadol), clonidine, iron tablets, diabetic medications (oral hypoglycaemics – lower blood sugar), and blood thinners (aspirin and warfarin) are dangerous if swallowed by a child
- discarded cigarette butts
- alcohol consumed by young children can lower brain glucose levels and cause brain damage

- inhaled solvents and glue sniffing cause seizures (fits), brain damage, hypoglycaemia (low blood sugar) and encephalopathy (brain inflammation)
- caustic household chemicals and household cleaning products containing bleach cause burns of the oesophagus if ingested
- oven cleaners if sprayed in the eyes can damage the corneas or cause vision loss

Choking

Choking on the following foods, especially when your child eats unsupervised in the car or in front of the TV, is a risk, especially in the first two years:
- big bits of carrot and celery
- grapes, cherry tomatoes and pieces of melon
- nuts, popcorn, corn chips and thick blobs of crunchy peanut butter
- hot dogs
- hard lollies and chewing gum

Other household hazards

- curtain cords can strangle or hang children and cause death by suffocation
- plastic bags can kill by suffocation if placed by a child over their head
- balloons can explode when bitten and be inhaled by a child and choke them
- laser pens and pointers directed at the eye can burn the retina (back part of the eye) and result in permanent loss of vision
- playing with matches or cigarette lighters can burn children and houses

- children unattended in the kitchen can sustain burns from pulling on overhanging oven pots or by touching hot oven elements or ceramic stovetops
- metal knives, forks or spoons in the electric toaster or power point can electrocute children
- hot cups of tea and coffee can scald and burn babies and young children so need to be consumed away from them
- small fingers can be trapped or cut off by hinged doors
- loose threads on a child's clothes can wrap around their fingers or toes and cut off their blood supply
- unsecured heavy items, like TV screens, heavy chests of drawers or garden decorations, can fall onto children if pulled and harm or even kill them
- basketball hoops attached to structures such as unstable garage walls can fall and crush children

Motor vehicles, boats, bikes and trolleys

- metal buckles on child seat restraints exposed to the sunlight get hot and can burn a child's skin
- slamming car doors on fingers can cut them off
- children and pets can die when left unattended in locked vehicles
- toddlers on the loose can be hit and killed by a reversing car in the driveway
- children without seatbelts or proper restraints in a vehicle are at high risk in the event of an accident
- children can sustain life-threatening head injuries if they don't wear a helmet on bikes and quad bikes
- falls from shopping trolleys can injure soft heads and break bones

Drownings and water hazards

- children can drown silently in unsecured pool areas
- defective pool gates allow children access to backyard pools
- toddlers can die at home if they trip and fall head first into a large laundry bucket of water
- children can die in baths
- burns can be sustained if the bath water is too hot
- babies can get hypothermic (very cold) in the swimming pool or ocean
- children can fall out of dinghies and be struck by the outboard motor propeller
- children without life jackets are placed at risk when boating
- ropes on boats can crush and cut off fingers and hands when pulled suddenly

Sun, heat and snow

- sunburn in babies and toddlers can result from even brief periods of sun exposure
- babies can die on the ski fields if exposed too long to harsh environmental conditions
- babies can get overheated in a spa

Farms

- beware the 'squishy' gum boot – this could be a frog or snake
- dams – drowning risk
- animals – dogs, horses and cows can injure children!
- snakes – venomous brown, tiger and dugite breeds
- industrial farm equipment
- tractors, cars, quad bikes and motorbikes
- petrol and chemicals
- firearms

- trees – falling branches
- bushfires
- isolation and difficulty of medical help and evacuation in an emergency

Animals
- poorly trained pets or aggressive dog breeds can bite, harm and kill young children
- falls from a horse or injury sustained from being kicked by a horse or cow
- birds, such as magpies, can swoop and attack a young child's eyes or face

Getting lost
- the child who becomes lost in a shopping centre is vulnerable to stranger danger
- the bush and outdoor areas can be dangerous for a child if they get lost, especially those with disability such as autism

Dental
- caries result when a young child falls asleep with a bottle of milk in their mouth

Allergy
- severe allergy, called anaphylaxis, affects breathing and can be caused by an allergy to nuts, such as peanuts, cashews, walnuts, almond and hazelnuts
- other allergies include egg, soy, wheat, seafood and shellfish
- grasses, bees and bull ants can cause severe allergic reactions

Part 4

Cruel friends

All about anxiety

Childhood anxiety is the most common childhood psychiatric disorder. Parents ask, 'Isn't anxiety normal in kids?' and 'Don't you mean "worry warts", "stress-ball kids" or lazy, manipulative students?' These are common misconceptions of childhood anxiety disorders.

As many as 1 in 5 children have anxiety symptoms and close to 1 in 30 have a generalised anxiety disorder (GAD). The American Psychiatric Association publishes a comprehensive reference text known as the *DSM-5*. It describes GADs as excessive, ongoing, insurmountable worries with physiological symptoms such as fast breathing and a rapid heart rate. These anxiety disorders impact on lifestyle and function and aren't explained by other medical conditions such as an overactive thyroid gland.

A little bit of anxiety helps, but a lot hinders. How we develop anxiety depends on the complex interplay between genetics, environment and neurobiological factors. This determines our brain's response to stressful situations. Our genes are implicated in the inheritance of anxiety traits in 30 to 50 per cent of cases of childhood anxiety. It's not our fault if we are anxious!

Anxious children can develop overwhelming anxiety and depression during adolescence and adulthood. The good news is that effective parenting practices modify anxiety. When they don't, your child could have an extra problem. This can be autism, ADHD, a learning disorder, depression or an eating disorder. It may indicate developmental trauma due to domestic violence – emotional, physical or sexual. Affected children and adults can present with long-term post-traumatic stress symptoms.

How does anxiety present?

This is the most common question I am asked about stressed-out kids and adolescents. The answer is best answered by recognising the many faces of this rising mental health condition.

Physiological symptoms

When you ask a child if they are worried or anxious, they deny this. Children don't always interpret the feeling of nausea, tummy aches, headaches, bad dreams, nail biting, 'butterflies in the stomach', avoidance or opting-out behaviours as anxiety. When you explain to them that some kids get scared of the dark or have bad dreams, they say, 'Yeah, that happens to me'.

Anxiety symptoms can include a rapid heart rate, palpitations, chest pain, shortness of breath, a sense of dread, fatigue, frequent urination, wetting, soiling, disturbed sleep, nightmares and constant fears. Worried children find it hard to concentrate and to complete school work. They complain of aches and pains.

'What if?' questions

The fearful and emotionally shaky child says, 'What if we have an accident on the way to school?' They ponder: 'What if mum doesn't come home?', 'My homework isn't finished', 'I will fail my test', 'No one wants to play with me' or 'Someone might break into the house and steal my toys'. They think: 'Monsters are hiding under my bed' or 'We could get attacked by terrorists'. Rational and irrational fears become blurred for the child who runs on high stress levels.

'Velcro kids'

These are young children who physically cling onto a parent. This is often their mother – they won't let go. These fearful kids hide under a chair or claw the carpet. They lack the emotional resilience to separate from their primary carer. This is more extreme than the normal separation anxiety seen in children starting school. If protracted, this emotional dysregulation may be due to autism.

Explosions

A parent sees the emotional dysregulation (temper tantrums) of the child and feels their distress. They are likely to absorb the intensity of the child's emotion and reflect it back upon the child. This perpetuates the cycle of worry and leads to the child internalising (imploding) or externalising (exploding) their anxiety.

Explosions occur in the form of emotional meltdowns. A child with pent-up feelings hits, punches, bites, screams, yells, throws objects or runs away. Parents become the external locus of a child's frustration and are physically attacked. A distraught child can grab a kitchen knife and threaten to cut you. Very anxious children will even threaten to kill themselves. They might place a rope around their neck or try to stab themselves with a knife or scissors. Children as young as 7 can initiate such actions.

If this happens you need to maintain calm. Overreacting will make things worse. Significant reactionary behaviour requires professional intervention. Timely preventive measures and an 'action plan' are preferable to families calling the police in crisis. But, some families are scared of their children and are forced to call the police or mental health crisis teams out of fear or for safety reasons.

Implosions

Some children cope with anxiety by emotionally shutting down and withdrawing socially and academically. They obsess, ruminate and have paranoid thoughts. They can be 'hearing voices' – usually the voice of anxiety. Rarely, this is a psychotic mental illness like schizophrenia.

The anxious child becomes quiet and non-communicative, regresses and retreats. They hide under school desks and chairs or in their bedroom. They lose interest in life and opt out of games, sports, extracurricular activities and learning.

Controlling and obsessive behaviours

Anxiety is contained by obsessive routines and controlling acts. Children restrict their dietary choices or stop eating. To maintain a sense of calm and be in charge, they will dictate the running of the home. These children tidy their rooms and the kitchen cupboards, sort out the linen and fastidiously clean the bathroom. Bugs, dirt and mess can become a fixation. They start to compulsively wash their hands and check that the lights are off or doors closed. This impairs their ability to do other things or even leave the house.

Oppositional behaviours

Obstinacy can develop when a child can't manage their anxiety. They feel out of control. These children become extremely stubborn and won't do what they are told by parents, teachers or outside people. Significant refusal to comply in a very young child can be seen in autism.

Avoidant actions

Evasive tactics are common in bright, anxious perfectionist kids. This cohort is strongly represented in children with high-functioning autism (HFA). When children sense they won't succeed, they become too scared to even try. If they are 'rescued' by an adult who enables them to avoid their fear, a maladaptive pattern of coping develops. A child refuses to do homework or attend school. They stop playing sport or participating in choir or drama activities. They have high performance and social anxiety and fail to reach their desired benchmark of perfection.

What makes anxiety worse?

This is a common query with a number of responses.

Anxious parents

The 'bounce' effect occurs when a child's fears are escalated by those of their parents and spread beyond the home and into the classroom and playground. Parents have to be the inert rock which absorbs the angst and not the mirror which reflects it back onto the child.

If you react to your child's anxiety with stress and indecision, your child can't remain calm. The same response occurs when anxious children have no limits set or are given too many choices. They will learn poor ways of coping with difficult situations. If parental anxiety becomes anger, a child can suffer from emotional and physical trauma and abuse.

Reactive responses
Becoming hysterical when your child is emotionally distraught only leads to bad choices being made. It exacerbates your child's anxiety. An example of this would be sending an impulsive email to your child's teacher at midnight. This is not a reflective or sensible action.

Inconsistent parenting
Inconsistent parenting makes a child feel insecure and unsafe. If a child never knows what response will result from their actions, they won't learn what is normal or expected behaviour.

Sibling rivalry
Conflict, tension, jealousy and competition between siblings escalates anxiety within households. It is more common when they are close in age and fighting for recognition in the same pursuits, such as sport, academic performance or music. If unresolved, it can result in emotional and physical abuse, severe anxiety, eating disorders and depression. Parental conflict and marital problems results. Timely professional advice is advised.

Overpraise
False affirmation doesn't teach or allow a child to learn through failure. To succeed they have to first fail a few times and build

emotional resilience. Then, they can 'have a go' and 'survive and thrive'.

Family breakdown

Marital discord can take the calm, reasonable and responsible out of parenting. Family stress elevates childhood anxiety. When parents split up they need to act as adults and sort out custodial issues as quickly as possible for the emotional safety of their child or children. Separation can be necessary to restore safety to households.

> One Saturday when browsing through the weekend papers I came across a chilling article. It showed the picture drawn by a child whose custodial care was shared between two households. She had drawn herself on a clock face. This was a powerful visual image from a child's perception that her fighting parents divided her life.

Family separation is a sad and emotive time for everyone involved. Many parents are able to put their differences aside and work together to provide certainty for their children. They make sure they practise consistent parenting. This provides the best family outcome. Children can be amazingly forgiving and adaptable. They can get used to a different routine, and find it is more calm than the turmoil prior to imminent separation.

Comorbid mental health problems

If anxiety is ignored during the early childhood years, it will resurface in later childhood, adolescence and early adult life. It appears as a generalised anxiety disorder, depression, eating disorder, obsessive-compulsive or oppositional defiant disorder.

Neurodevelopmental conditions

Anxiety often accompanies and complicates ADHD and SLDs. It unmasks autism and makes it worse. Children who function at a high level with autism can have a normal façade but retain great emotional fragility. Their anxiety often translates into depression as they transition towards the teenage years.

What can a parent do?

Small steps taken by loving parents and families early in a child's life can make a difference. It is never too late to try, even if you are faced with a fearful and sad teenager. If you need help, speak with your doctor, social worker, school counsellor or a clinical psychologist. The following 'tips' point you in the right direction to seek the appropriate help for your needs. I expand on them throughout the relevant text in each of the childhood age groups.

Read the behaviour of your child

Your anxious child is sending you a message. A meltdown is saying, 'I am overwhelmed and I need your help'. The out-of-control young child is not a 'naughty' child.

Acknowledge your anxious child

It is not helpful to say, 'Don't worry'. Your child or teenager is scared, anxious and very worried. They need you to recognise this and take charge as an adult.

Wait for calm

To help an anxious child you have to be 'still' yourself. Parenting is most effective when both the child and parent are calm. Normal parenting techniques don't work when a toddler or adolescent is having a major 'wobbly'. Reflect and act as a support person, to guide and mentor. You can't fix your child's problems. They have to learn how to do this. You won't always be around to 'rescue' them.

Firm but fair rules and boundaries

When parents take charge and provide calm, consistent guidelines for children, they provide a safety net for anxious children. Flexibility has to be retained as rigid and controlling parenting can be harmful and even emotionally abusive. It results in heightened anxiety in children and oppositional responses.

Family stability

Consider the needs of all family members. This enables your family to stay strong. Limit the busyness in your life. Take time to walk, talk and be active. Monitor and supervise electronic screen time. Reconnect with extended family members. Talk to neighbours.

Unconditional love

It's alright to love your child unconditionally, but don't smother them with love. This will prevent them from growing emotional and social resilience.

Teach your child to fail

You can never be a perfect parent. But keep trying to be the best parent you can. Show your children your imperfections and how you deal with them. This teaches them helpful coping strategies.

Don't rescue your child

Stand up to anxiety. Work out ways with your child to be the 'boss' of their worries. If you step in to solve your child's problems, they won't learn ways to do this themselves. Raise your child to be an independent, confident and emotionally strong young adult.

Rationalise fears

Help your child understand the difference between real fears and irrational ones. Dinosaurs falling from the sky and squashing your car is an unrealistic worry. Hurting yourself by diving from a 10-metre diving board when you haven't dived before is a healthy fear.

Decrease a child's sensory load

Don't drag your emotionally intense toddler to the shops at peak times. This is relevant if your child has autism. They find loud sounds, bright lights, strong smells and certain textures and textiles physically and emotionally painful.

Limit setting

This helps the performance pressure of timed tasks and assessments. Tell a child they only have to write one page of work each day or perform two tasks. This defines and contains their 'chores' and keeps them manageable. It allows a child to succeed at something and to engage with learning. Make sure you set the 'bar of expectation' at a manageable height for the age and stage of your child.

Minimal choices

Having only one or two choices reduces the anxiety of decision-making. Always telling your child what to do leads to rigid parenting. Children will oppose this style of discipline. If you give your child two manageable options, you allow them to be in control. This makes them feel secure. Say, for example, 'Do you want to watch *Toy Story* or *Frozen*?' If they can't decide, then you make the decision and stick to it. Don't ask, 'Which DVD do you want to see?' With anxious young children, parents have to be in charge.

Who can help?

There are many people and numerous resources to help families, teachers and mentors assist an anxious child. A compassion-focused approach is a good start. Fretful and stressed children require great patience, nurture and kindness.

Parental mental health

Address your own anxiety or depression before trying to support your anxious child. You must be calm to keep your child calm. If you are medically unfit or have untreated adult ADHD, it can be hard to achieve this. Seek help from your local doctor, psychiatrist or psychologist.

Professional help

Contact your child health nurse, local doctor, paediatrician, child and adolescent psychiatrist, clinical psychologist, social worker and your child's teachers. Allied health professionals, such as occupational therapists, speech pathologists and physiotherapists, also have an important role. Never be too proud or afraid to ask for help.

Connect with community

When you help others you will find yourself well supported. You will feel happier.

Medications

Children need medication when they have overwhelming and debilitating anxiety or depression. Medication can stabilise their mood. This allows adjunctive treatments, including intense and ongoing psychological and psychiatric counselling, to be effective.

Two main types of medication help anxious, angry and sad children. They are called selective serotonin reuptake inhibitors (SSRIs) and atypical antipsychotics. I mention them briefly. Your child is unlikely to require them.

The two most commonly prescribed SSRIs in children are fluoxetine and sertraline. You might recognise these drugs as Prozac and Zoloft. They work by increasing the level of serotonin, a mood chemical, naturally produced by the body. In children under 18 years of age they are not formally approved and are prescribed as 'off label'. This is legal.

Risperidone is an atypical antipsychotic class of medication approved for the medical management of severe aggression and anxiety in children with autism. Aripiprazole or Abilify is another. Medical specialists prescribe these potent medications.

Parents ask whether to give the herbal preparation St John's wort to their depressed or anxious child. It is not recommended in children and may increase the side effects of some medications such as SSRIs.

We treat debilitating anxiety and depression in adults, so why should children be excluded from medical treatment when it can make a difference? Mental ill health is a medical condition, just as important as physical disease. Mental distress is a recent term. It describes the pain of this illness for the victim and their families.

For some children medication is a last resort. It can help them function, attend school and learn. More importantly, it can help them connect and socialise with their peers rather than remain sad and withdrawn. If children are debilitated by severe anxiety, they refuse to go to school and fall further behind academically. They are ostracised by their classmates and other parents.

Parental consent

Discussion about the use and potential side effects of medications for anxiety is required before they are prescribed. Consent to treat a child with anti-anxiety medication should be from both parents, especially in cases of family separation. Medicating children is a traumatic decision for families. Families should not be judged for the actions they take to help their child.

Other supports

Prescription drugs should never be given in isolation. Input is required with paediatricians, family doctors, psychiatrists, psychologists and therapists. Parents and schools also need to be on board.

Anxiety and comorbid mental health disorders can be overwhelming, but are often seen in awesome, creative and clever people. It is helpful to see the needs of people rather than their diagnosis. This is the best way to respect, understand and enjoy their company.

You can cope with an anxious child if you invite humour, resolve, patience, humility and resilience to share your journey. The skills and strategies you learn together to deal with adversity such as anxiety and depression will make your family stronger. You will learn tolerance and compassion. Adversity restores perspective.

There are a number of references, texts and online resources relating to anxiety cited at the end of this book.

Anxiety – 0 to 5 years

Childhood anxiety often starts with anxious mothers and fathers and their high aspirations of parenthood.

Unrealistic expectations

Rigid birthing plans and fictional feed and sleep schedules place unrealistic expectations on parenting. They are a recipe for failure.

Babies are born anxious

Babies are exposed to a biologically stressed environment when their mothers are anxious, depressed or take illicit or certain classes of prescribed medications. A mother can be the victim of domestic violence, mental distress or addiction. She needs medical and family support, not judgement. Her baby may have symptoms of drug withdrawal when born. These babies react to their adverse environment by becoming hyperaroused, fretful and tense. They are overtired and feed and sleep poorly. This makes a fatigued mother feel inadequate. She then struggles to bond and form a healthy attachment to her baby.

Anxious households

As many as 1 in 6 women in our country are physically or sexually abused by their partner. Their children witness adversity and become victims of developmental trauma. Children sense fear and conflict, even from a young age. They smell it. They learn to read the signs of anxiety and concern from the posture, gestures, facial expressions and tone of their parents' voices. They show distress by becoming quiet and withdrawn or act out with physical aggression. Their mood is labile. When they start school they appear inattentive and distracted.

Maternal–infant bonding

The importance of the secure, emotional attachment of an infant to its mother is a relatively recent epiphany. It sets the scene for building emotionally strong and resilient children.

Parenting styles have a critical role in determining whether a child becomes anxious. Inconsistent nurturing leads to disorganised and chaotic attachment between a child and parent. This creates anxiety.

If a baby cries it may be hungry, cold, tired, bored, or just have a dirty nappy. If their cry is heard and their needs attended to, they will be reassured and settle. If the response to their cry is uncertain they become fearful or agitated.

Settling your anxious baby

Some babies are born laid-back and others, even in calm arms, are agitated and unhappy. If you have one of these 'jumping bean' babies, you will need to take turns at settling your baby.

Some mothers feel a sense of failure when they can't quiet their distressed baby. Self-esteem dives when their partner or a friend takes over and their baby instantly ceases to cry. This is normal. Sit down, have a cup of tea or coffee and enjoy a few moments to yourself. Don't reach for a wine!

Sometimes babies get overtired. If you think about your own reactions in this state it can be hard to fall asleep. You need to read your baby's 'tired' signs. Hold them close. Pat, but never shake, them and gently rock your baby before placing them on their back in their cot. It is important to practise consistent and repetitive settling techniques with your baby so that they develop a good sleep pattern in their first 12 months.

Child health nurses give practical advice about settling techniques. Support and centres such as Ngala in WA and

Tresillian Family Care Centres in NSW provide excellent online and phone advice, consultation and the opportunity for overnight observational stays if your baby is not sleeping. Other states have similar support services. These contact details are readily sourced online.

Separation anxiety

You need some attachment to your child in the same way as a bungee jumper depends on their rope. The rope shouldn't be too tight or too slack. In the same way, you don't want the attachment to your child and toddler to be so dependent that they have difficulty separating from you.

Some clinginess is normal when children first start school. Teachers are helpful in assisting parents and children with this milestone. Many children take a transitional object to school such as a soft toy. 'Mr Rabbit' or 'Bear' is their safety rope between the security and familiarity of home and the strangeness of school. The anxious or emotionally insecure child becomes overly dependent on this 'prop'.

Your child may cling to your side and cry inconsolably when you drop them off at kindergarten. Some children separate too easily. They are happy to go to anyone for comfort. Get this balance right and your child will cope with the separations necessary as they progress through childhood, and so will you.

Separation anxiety that is pervasive, persistent and severe requires intervention with a clinical psychologist, paediatrician or child psychiatrist. It can indicate autism.

Selective mutism

This is a severe form of social anxiety. It is situational and driven by paralysing anxiety. A child with this diagnosis may not speak in public or to another person such as a doctor or teacher. They whisper to a parent in front of you. They may stay silent but speak more freely to family. Sometimes a child will only speak to one person, usually their mother. It can be difficult to separate this condition from autism, especially high functioning autism. Selective mutism commonly starts around the age of 2 to 4 years.

It is important to work proactively with these kids and their parents. An experienced clinical psychologist and a child psychiatrist or paediatrician evaluates the nature of the maternal–child bond. In severe cases, an SSRI medication for anxiety is prescribed.

Common fears

Fear of the dark is normal if you are 4 years old. If it persists and remains unresolved it becomes maladaptive and impacts on a family's sleep routine. Anxiety is not just an adult affliction. The 4-year-old child can experience fear, hopelessness and despair. They are afraid of becoming lost or their parents going away. Three year olds can be frightened of lifts and the 4-year-old child scared of tackling stairs. Children can suffer from mental distress.

The management of childhood anxiety

Anxious children need routine, structure and adequate preparation and notification of their daily timetable. They don't cope with rush, panic and changeability. They do best with minimal choices and defined end points.

If you want to help your anxious child you have to first manage your own emotions, mood swings, sadness and anxieties.

Note your young child's worries but refrain from keeping them on board. You can't fix everything. Try not to 'rescue' the anxious child. Your child needs to learn how to face fear and failure with the knowledge that you are there to help.

Doing your child's shoelaces up every time won't teach them how to do their 'bunny ears'. Do you want your teenager wearing sneakers with velcro straps? If you do, then keep tying their laces.

Fail to recognise the language of your distraught child and you will have to manage their emotional meltdown. The toddler and young child will kick, punch, throw, bang, bite, scream and run. Young children need a physical outlet for pent-up emotions. To interrupt them while they off-load their rage is not helpful. Work on reading the triggers and warning signs to prevent the meltdown. Assist with strategies to limit them.

Normal parenting strategies do not work when a child is having a major tantrum. You have to make sure that your child is safe, step back and wait until the storm has passed.

Acknowledge your child's distress. They are often embarrassed. This creates further trauma for them, particularly with public displays of 'poor behaviour'.

Suggest some ways that they can control their fears and anger so that they don't become big worries. It doesn't help to dwell on what has passed.

Young children can identify what makes them 'mad'. When calm they will listen to your suggestions or to those made by a clinical psychologist, school psychologist, counsellor, teacher or doctor.

Help your child recognise their weaknesses, encourage their strengths and teach them to learn through failure. This way you will give them skills to protect their mental health for life.

The consequence of childhood anxiety

Small worries in a child become greater worries during their later childhood and teen years. Anxious children get more stressed, obsessive, aggressive or depressed during adolescence if they don't have the emotional resilience to cope with puberty and social change. The early childhood years are the time to get the recipe of raising children nearly right. If you can't do this, you will struggle through later childhood and adolescence.

Timely management of anxiety is preventive and protective against later adolescent and adult mental health problems. Instituted early, it is a worthwhile and cost-efficient investment in our children.

Anxiety – 5 to 10 years

The rise of anxiety is the consequence of our altered social climate and unrealistic aspirations. Anxiety pervades every stage of childhood. It is a great chameleon. During the early school years, anxiety presents as separation anxiety; emotional dysregulation or 'meltdowns'; sleep disturbance; panic attacks; phobias; and social anxiety, including selective mutism. It results in school avoidance and school non-attendance. Anxiety makes autism worse and the effects of bullying more powerful. It is a recognised comorbid mental health condition, linked with ADHD, autism, learning problems and eating disorders. Unresolved, it leads to adolescent and adult mental health conditions of GAD, depression and self-harm.

Separation anxiety

This is an emotional state of excessive clinginess and reluctance to separate from a parent in social situations such as school. In very young children this fear is an understandable reaction when facing the unknown without the security of mum or dad. It can be normal for a child's developmental stage. First days at day care or kindergarten are likely to evoke this emotion.

It is abnormal when it is exaggerated, persistent and insurmountable. Children with autism and anxiety are the most likely to display early, persistent and pervasive separation anxiety.

Learning to leave a parent in the knowledge that the parent will return allows a child to achieve independence. To assist their child through this transition a parent should appear confident and in control. If you can leave your child at school with reassuring words and a calm demeanour, your child is more likely to mirror your feelings. If your reaction is of fear, sadness, agitation or uncertainty, then your child will amplify these emotions.

Early school non-attendance

During the early school years there will be days when your child wants to stay home. They complain of tiredness. That their tummy or head hurts. Most parents are quick to keep their child at home. Parents know their child best. I would not dispute their decision, but it is important that parents don't enable a pattern of early school avoidance.

One of my friends permitted sick days, but her children stayed in bed. They were well looked after, could read and do school work, but had no electronic screen privileges. If they were sick they didn't complain.

If children avoid school, parents need to ask the child about who they play with at lunchtime. Is schoolwork too easy, too hard or just right? Parents need to speak with the teacher for feedback. Has their child been bullied and traumatised?

One child I cared for had spiteful graffiti written about her on the toilet doors at school. The handwriting was readily identifiable, but the deputy principal dismissed the child's victimisation by simply washing off the

*offensive text. The child was only in year 3. She had already been
ostracised by her peer group. She had started running away from school
when dropped off.*

When a child is emotionally distressed we must listen to their
cries and advocate for the child. I would support a family removing
their young child from this unfavourable social setting because it
is unlikely to change for that child.

Specific fears or phobias

These can be triggered by a single event, perceived as emotionally
traumatic by the child. A young child bitten by a dog may later panic
at the sight of one. They avoid going to parks in case they see a dog.
Sometimes the trigger for a child's extreme anxiety is unknown.

If your child develops a phobia, intervene quickly to overcome
it. Do this with help from an experienced clinical psychologist.
Severe or resistant phobias need input from a child psychiatrist.

You can't reason or dismiss a child's fears. You have to work
with the child to get them to face their fears and resolve their
problems.

Emotional meltdowns

Your child may display their worries and frustrations by screaming,
crying, shouting, kicking or punching. You can't 'fix' your child's
tantrum. Wait until they have calmed down. Give them plenty of
space so that they don't feel trapped. If you try to hold them, they
will kick and punch even more.

Restraining the screaming child in a school situation is not
helpful. It reinforces the trauma a child experiences.

Domestic violence

It is an adult responsibility to protect and nurture our children. They have the right to a safe home and a good education. Children need to be well cared for physically and emotionally. When this doesn't happen, they become the victims of developmental trauma. Anxiety is one of the presentations of adverse childhood events such as emotional or sexual abuse. Doctors, parents and teachers must consider this possibility.

Medical conditions

Abdominal pain is one of the most common childhood complaints. When it occurs in conjunction with a headache and pallor it is often called an 'abdominal migraine'. Mostly it resolves. Anxiety is often attributed as a cause of chronic abdominal pain of childhood. It is still important to exclude medical and surgical problems.

Sleep and other problems

The anxious child has problems sleeping in their own bed. They seek reassurance about the safety of their room and get parents to check for monsters or bad people. Parents dread the night-time ritual of saying goodnight because it takes three hours instead of twenty minutes. The parent, often the mother, will do everything she can to keep the home calm and running. The child ends up sleeping with parents or a parent sleeps in the child's room.

This causes sleep deprivation and high stress levels to build within the home. Bit by bit, the family starts to implode and a high-anxiety state is created.

Maintaining a healthy eating, work, play and sleep cycle can help. If a child is physically tired they sleep better. A night-time story and talk time helps. Watching violent or scary movies before bed won't. Limiting access to electronic devices around bedtime is essential.

Persistent sleep disturbance due to anxiety benefits from help provided by a clinical psychologist.

Bullying

Some kids don't like school. Someone is mean, the teacher screams or no one will play with them. Cyberbullying has become part of primary school culture. Children with autism and anxious children are particularly vulnerable to being socially ostracised. This is a form of bullying.

Bullying can make children worried and sad. Parents need to be attuned to their child's moods and be ready to listen when they ask for help. Children don't always ask for help at the most convenient times but be glad when they do.

Schools are now expected to have effective anti-bullying policies in place to combat cyberbullying, and social, emotional and physical bullying. They have to report the inappropriate use of social media and electronic devices as an electronic breach – an e-breach. If they fail to act upon bullying complaints and a student's mental health is compromised, they can be held liable.

Children are being empowered to stand up to bullies. They understand that children who bully have their own insecurities. The Alannah and Madeline Foundation, a national charity set up to protect children from violence, encourages children to maintain a firm stance against bullies. The National Centre Against Bullying (NCAB) assists schools and communities to address physical, emotional and cyberbullying.

Autism and bullying

Peer conformity at school still dictates social acceptance and makes it difficult for children with autism to fit in. The child with autism who has expertise with Lego blocks, *Club Penguin, Minecraft* or *Pokémon* is accepted by their peers in primary school. Transition to the socially diverse environment of high school is difficult. They face bullying unless they move with a supportive primary school cohort, or channel their focus into electronic gaming or computer and technology expertise. They are then respected as computer nerds. Children with autism have as much right to belong in their school as any other child.

Fighting bullies

Most schools have a zero tolerance policy towards bullying. They provide good resources to acknowledge and help the child who is bullied.

If bullying is relentless, a child and their family benefit from speaking with a clinical psychologist for several sessions. I explain to kids that psychologists are good at listening. They suggest great ways of feeling strong and confident. This helps to deal with worries.

There are some great books on bullying that help kids. These include the *I Am Jack* series by Susanne Gervay and *Beating the Bullies* by Dr Lucy Blunt.

Further resources on bullying are listed in the 'Helpful reading' section.

Quiet worriers

Watch out for the secret worrier. This describes the child who withdraws socially and academically and is hard to re-engage.

They don't ask for help. This happens with very intuitive, bright children who overthink life. They tend to be perfectionists who fail to keep up with the high goals they have set themselves as they progress through school.

You see this in children with high functioning autism. They internalise their anxiety and then they become depressed. Or, they develop obsessive and controlling behaviours in an attempt to contain their anxiety. In this cohort, anxiety starts as a subtle change, but if ignored can have a devastating impact on the child and their family. Ask for professional help early if your child falls into this group.

Anxiety and autism

Anxiety is poorly understood in children with autism. Children with high functioning autism who are doing well academically in the primary school years can present with a normal façade. Teachers and family think that they are all right when they're not. Kids who are good at drama, very bright students and the anxious perfectionist can also mask their symptoms well.

Anxiety and depression is often missed in these children.

What can children do?

It is best for anxious children to off-load big worries on mums and dads. Young kids can paint a shoebox, make a slot in the lid and post a worry each night. They store their box of worries under mum and dad's bed. Anxious children understand this concept. It may not work for the very bright or logical child.

Most kids work well with a clinical psychologist to break down worries into manageable packages. By doing this, they experience success. This provides incentive to tackle other problems. They learn how to read their anxiety symptoms and control them; to slow down their breathing, be mindful of their emotions and take 'sensory breaks'. This removes them from the hectic pace of the classroom.

What can parents do?

If your child is worried, anxious and fearful, you have to take notice and act. Listen to your child. Speak with your partner and think carefully about how you are going to approach the problem. First, acknowledge your child's anxiety. You can then work out some strategies for them to deal with it. Let them know that you are there to help.

You can't 'fix' anxious behaviours. As your child grows they will have to develop greater independence which includes working out their own strategies to face fears.

If your child has an anxious personality, it helps to pick them up from school at least once during the week. Talk with your employer about a flexi-day so that you can maintain connectivity with your child at school. This allows you to observe your child's body language at the end of the day. You can see if they are happy and playing with other kids. Speak with the other parents and work out who are your child's friends. It is helpful to establish this in the primary school years because you don't get to meet other parents as easily in the high school years.

Children who are being relentlessly bullied need adult help. Believe your child when they say they are being bullied. Avoid over-reacting. Act proportionately and appropriately. Get a psychologist involved, notify the school. In severe cases, contact the police.

A proactive approach is needed to intercept early childhood anxiety and to prevent problematic childhood and adolescent anxiety disorders.

You are not a bad or overreactive parent if you seek help early for your very anxious child. If you seek help for yourself, you are an even better parent.

Help can come from family, friends or neighbours, teachers, the school nurse, school psychologist or counsellor. Your family doctor may refer you to a psychologist, paediatrician or child psychiatrist. Do what you have to do to address the needs of your child, your family and yourself. Adopt a sensible and proportionate response to your child's problem.

Anxiety – 10 to 15 years

Teenage anxiety is most problematic when we fail to recognise and act aggressively to manage early childhood anxiety. Many parents out of love try to rescue, protect and hover over the anxious infant and young child, who then becomes an anxious older child. They inadvertently smother the emotional development of their child. Parents can mirror and amplify their child's anxiety, particularly if they are struggling with feelings of isolation, desperation, anxiety and depression.

The emerging adolescent with anxiety needs a compassion-focused approach by parents and teachers. Academic and social anxiety, school non-attendance, adjusting to pubertal change and mental health comorbidity are the main causes of anxiety in the initial high school years. Anxiety makes autism significantly worse in this age group.

School disengagement

Failure to attend school occurs in any of the high school years. It becomes a significant problem once students are in years 9 and 10 as it impacts on their chances to complete school.

Students are well supported in primary school because of the tight structure of their classroom and support of their peer group but don't cope with the social anxiety and performance pressure of secondary school. The academic workload becomes more onerous from year 9.

Kids with specific learning disorders such as dysgraphia and dyslexia often disengage from learning. They sense that they have already failed school and opt out of the traditional education system. Students most affected are those with a generalised anxiety disorder, high functioning autism, ADHD, depression or an eating disorder. These are the kids who tend to be intuitive 'over-thinkers', perfectionists, or intellectually gifted with high academic goals.

School disengagement occurs when a student is severely traumatised by the school system's social and academic expectations. It is the consequence of mental health complexity, compounded by family and individual factors. Tertiary intervention is nearly always required with a team of mental healthcare professionals. A child and adolescent psychiatrist and clinical psychologist are essential but the family and school remain the linchpins and best support the emerging adolescent.

Anxiety and autism

Anxious children are extremely sensitive about their behaviour – often ashamed and remorseful. They need understanding, patience, tolerance and their privacy respected. When you are the parent of a child with significant emotional needs, refrain from discussing them within earshot of the child.

The mother of a 14-year-old boy told me how difficult he was, especially in the mornings when he would shout and scream. She stated that his bad behaviour was affecting the whole family. Her son bravely stated that he agreed with her but requested that she not tell his grandmother over the phone how awful he was. He described feeling too embarrassed to speak with his grandmother, knowing that his bad behaviours had been discussed with her. How would you feel as a parent if your child shared your bad moods, behaviours or alcohol consumption with your colleagues, family or friends?

If you are the parent of a child with many needs, you may have to share your burden of emotional duress. Think carefully about how and when you do this. Seek help and support for yourself outside the family or your friendship circle so that you can remain strong to deal with the significant load of a child battling with anxiety or depression.

Help can be sought from a clinical psychologist, counsellor or medical doctor. There are also times when it is appropriate to speak initially with close family or an understanding friend or colleague. Take care not to blur the boundaries of friendship and counselling. You can lose your friend. Friendships are best kept positive.

Anxiety and autism are close friends and if not monitored become autism and depression during the vulnerable pre-adolescent and adolescent years of 11 to 15 years. This is when the structure and social scaffolding of the primary school years is replaced by too much flexibility and choice. During the high school years anxious children still require firm boundaries and limited options.

Anxiety and depression are often missed during this vulnerable time, even by paediatricians and child and adolescent psychiatrists. We don't always recognise the salient progression of social and academic withdrawal during the early high school years and the retreat of the child's personality into a protective shell due to depression.

As professionals we need to heed the words and wisdom of wise mentors who share their knowledge and experience with us. We have to recognise mental health problems and their triggers earlier.

All about autism spectrum disorder (ASD)

What is autism?

Autism is a neurodevelopmental disorder diagnosed from as early as 2 to 4 years of age. Autism can occasionally be diagnosed prior to the age of 2 years. Diagnosis can be delayed until later childhood or adolescence. In this condition the brain thinks differently. Children develop with atypical childhood language patterns, social and behavioural milestones. Children who don't have autism are often called 'neurotypicals'.

Language problems

Children with autism have problems with the development and use of spoken and unspoken language to communicate with meaning and understanding. They have language delay, don't speak at all or talk in stilted phrases. Children with no or minimal language are described as nonverbal. Social phrases are echolalic (repetitive), rehearsed or stereotypic. The child with autism may only use learned phrases such as 'How are you today?' when greeting someone. A prompt (reminder) is needed to elicit this welcome.

Social problems

Autism is associated with children who have poor eye contact and gaze aversion – they look away when spoken to. They find it hard to start a conversation and appear socially awkward within their peer group. Rich, symbolic, imaginative or pretend play can be deficient. These kids have problems with joint attention (showing and sharing), joining in and social situations. Friendships are hard to make or are restricted to clinging on to a socially competent peer.

Theory of mind

Autism can displace empathy from a child's perspective of the world. The concept of 'theory of mind' develops around 4 to 5 years in most children. This term describes how we understand the thoughts and emotions of others. It is impaired in children with ASD. They have problems 'walking in someone else's shoes' and don't 'get' social context.

Social aloofness doesn't equate with a lack of compassion. Children with autism just have a logical, practical and fair way of viewing life. They can be loving and caring, especially within family units.

High functioning autism

High functioning autism (HFA) is characterised by normal or advanced language development. It is often understood as Asperger syndrome. These children have good cognitive intelligence but struggle with social and emotional intelligence. This means they have problems reading social cues and make frequent gaffes. It is hard to find friends who understand them.

Their language can be eloquent with an extensive vocabulary. They can adopt an accent or affected conversational voice. Kids with HFA can be quirky and creative but also literal and concrete in their thought processes. A spade is a spade – it can't be a shovel!

The blunt use of language can result in an autistic child appearing rude and abrupt. They might point out the pimple on your nose or tell you that you are fat, both of which will be correct.

> *After consulting with a 12-year-old boy who has high functioning autism, the boy in a matter-of-fact tone said, 'Enjoy your monetary fee now'. His parents were embarrassed, but I understood the intent of his comment. It was warm-hearted.*

The child with high functioning autism with Asperger presentation perseverates on topics on which they have vast knowledge. If this is on a socially 'cool' topic, they are respected. But when the primary school student is still immersed in the virtual world of Club Penguin or Minecraft when they transition to high school, they can be socially ostracised.

Behavioural problems

Sensory and behavioural problems are common in autism. Loud sounds, bright lights, strong smells, tactile sensations from clothes and certain food textures can overwhelm the child with autism. These sensory 'insults' are excruciatingly painful and can precipitate a 'meltdown'.

> *A boy with autism explained that when his mother bit into a chip, he had to place his hands over his ears because the sound she made was extraordinarily loud and annoying to him.*

The child with autism controls their emotions by becoming sensory seeking. They show 'stimming' behaviours which include fixated and repetitive actions such as flicking, rocking, twirling, hand flapping and head banging.

They develop obsessive behaviours, rituals and routines evident by restricted and selective food intake, clothes choices and rigid and limited play. Repetitive behaviours seen in autism include lining up and stacking objects, preferences for specific colours, shapes or numbers, and fixations on moving objects such as fans or water.

Early presentation

Autism presents early because of lack of language and social development. Classically, autism is seen in the infant and young child who starts to develop normally but then stagnates or loses language milestones. Parents report that their child was smiling and had a couple of words in the first 12 months of life, but then became quiet, withdrawn and stopped speaking at around 11 to 20 months of life. Some parents will recall subtle changes from 6 to 9 months, before their child's 12-month immunisations.

They describe difficulties bonding with their infant because they were always irritable, hypervigilant, tense, fed poorly and seemed detached. Mothers who give this history can have a history of postnatal depression and an attachment disorder. But, sometimes these early difficulties indicate autism.

Later presentation

Severe separation anxiety and persistent dysregulated behaviours manifest by prolonged and severe tantrums in early childhood can be part of the autism spectrum disorders. These behaviours can be misinterpreted as 'naughty' children or ADHD.

High functioning autism can present during the vulnerable early high school years when a child is 11 to 15 years of age.

Academic performance and social function decline. This cohort present with severe anxiety, school avoidance and refusal, social withdrawal, chronic fatigue and depression. They disengage from school, learning and extracurricular activities.

The very bright child masks their autism symptoms until the social anxiety of the later school years causes them to decompensate emotionally, socially and academically.

Autism is often accompanied and complicated by ADHD, anxiety, depression and learning disorders. This can complicate its diagnosis during the teenage years.

The young adult with missed high functioning autism can fail when they enter the tertiary education system. Generally, they become overwhelmed by social and academic performance pressures and get depressed. They opt out of social activities and can become reclusive. Social media can be a lifeline for them.

The many faces of autism

Parents fear autism despite greater public awareness and under-standing of how autism can affect children. Education has demystified much of what autism is and is not, but parents still associate it with savant qualities. These are splinter skills of extra-ordinary ability. In the 1988 movie *Rain Man*, the actor Dustin Hoffman plays a savant with an exceptional memory for statistics and counting cards.

Tim Sharp is an international artist and creator of the superhero Laser Man. He also has autism.

In the popular US sitcom *The Big Bang Theory,* Jim Parsons plays the character of Sheldon, a nerdy scientist who gets himself into a number of social dilemmas. He displays a number of the social skills difficulties experienced in Asperger syndrome.

Autism is labelled a spectrum disorder because of its hetero-geneity. The child immersed in his own world, unable to talk or communicate and displaying sensory-seeking behaviours such as sniffing, hand flapping, spinning, rocking and headbanging can have autism. So too can the bright child who fabricates an elaborate fantasy world of imaginary friends or fantasy characters to be their social haven. In adolescence, the equivalent is connectivity with virtual friends which replaces the need for face-to-face friendships.

How is autism diagnosed?

The *DSM-5* is used in Australia to diagnose autism. States and territories have different diagnostic standards. National guide-lines are being proposed to standardise autism diagnosis. Western Australia is recognised as having high clinical standards for autism assessment. A multidisciplinary opinion is provided by a paedia-trician or psychiatrist, clinical psychologist and speech pathologist. In children over 12 years of age, a diagnosis can be made by a clinical psychologist and paediatrician or psychiatrist. Assessments are provided in both the private and public health sectors. Referral to a medical specialist is made by the family doctor. Information about a child's learning, socialisation and development is also requested from educators and the child's family.

DSM-5 *criteria*

The *DSM-5* classification requires 'persistent deficits in social communication and social interaction across multiple contexts'. Three social criteria must be evident at presentation or described historically from early childhood. These are problems with social–emotional reciprocity, nonverbal communication and peer relationships. This means difficulties in talking and participating in a social setting, poor use of eye contact, misinterpretation of social cues and lack of imaginative play and reciprocal friendships.

In addition, at least two out of four listed 'restricted, repetitive patterns of behaviour, interests or activities' have to be met to a level of severity that affects a child's daily function. These can be repetitive and stereotypic motor movements such as lining up objects, tiptoe walking or hand flapping. Pedantic, ritualistic routines, the fear of changing how things are done, fixated and obsessive interests and unusual sensory reactivity constitute the other areas.

Autistic traits have to occur in multiple settings and not be explained by intellectual disability. This means that a child can have autism and a low IQ but their behaviour can't be attributed solely to their intellectual deficit.

It is easy to look up the *DSM-5* criteria for autism online, but the interpretation needs the expertise of clinicians. It can be difficult even for trained professionals to distinguish between autism, significant language disorder, ADHD, intellectual disability, severe anxiety, profound hearing loss and emotionally traumatised children. That's why a multidisciplinary diagnostic approach is necessary.

DSM-5 criteria does not include Asperger syndrome or PDD-NOS (pervasive development disorder, not otherwise specified), sometimes referred to as atypical autism. Children previously diagnosed with these disorders under earlier *DSM-IV* criteria retain a diagnosis of ASD.

Asperger

The new *DSM-5* criteria for autism excludes some children who in the past would have met a diagnosis of Asperger. People with Asperger syndrome who call themselves 'Aspies' feel their identity was stolen when the new classification for autism was introduced. Some of these children will meet the criteria for HFA.

Pathological demand avoidance

An emerging subtype of autism is pathological demand avoidance (PDA) syndrome. This describes children who meet criteria for an autism spectrum disorder but have extreme obstinacy and reluctance to comply. Much of their presentation is driven by high anxiety and the need to be in control. This further increases anxiety and leads to obsessive behaviours, often directed towards familiar people. Sometimes this syndrome is attributed to discordant parenting and dysfunctional families.

This pattern of behaviour becomes problematic from early adolescence when children with high functioning autism demonstrate increased avoidance patterns of behaviour. This relates to certain social situations or to school. It is a very complex variant of autism to manage.

A similar clinical picture, characterised by social withdrawal and determined resistance to treatment, has been described in the literature as pervasive refusal syndrome. It is described as occurring particularly in girls with genetic vulnerability from age 8 to 15 years and is thought to be precipitated by an infection or incidental injury.

Screening tools

A number of autism screening materials and apps are used by parents, teachers and health professionals to detect the early presentation of autism.

It is beyond the scope of this book to discuss these screening devices. Parents, families, child health nurses and teachers are often the best guide as to which children should be assessed for autism.

How many children have autism?

Since the 1990s, an increased number of children globally have been diagnosed with ASD. The rise is exponential. The number of children diagnosed appears to be doubling every three years. The predicted final rate of autism diagnosis in Australia for the year 2015 was reported to be 230,000. This raises the query: 'Is autism being over-diagnosed?' This is relevant for the sustainability of Australia's National Disability Insurance Scheme (NDIS) to adequately fund for autism.

The prevalence of autism varies from 1 in 50 to 1 in 500. In the US, some figures quote 1 in 68 children as having autism.

The accepted incidence is around 1 in 100. Exact figures for the prevalence of autism are not available.

Boys are four times more likely to be diagnosed with ASD than girls. I think we miss a number of teenage girls with high functioning autism with Asperger features. This is because girls tend to be more social in their play from an early age compared with boys.

An intelligent girl with Asperger is often mentored by a socially competent friend and so learns to read the social cues from observation. They engage more in social activities such as drama.

'Is the increase in autism real, or are we diagnosing children to facilitate funding and access to early intervention services?' There is a risk of this condition being 'over diagnosed', but my clinical experience is that autism is on the rise.

One of the reasons for this observation is that the rate of childhood anxiety is climbing. Anxiety increases the prevalence of autism because it unmasks its symptoms. It makes autism worse.

Autism in families

Families who already have one child with autism have a risk of around 10 per cent of subsequent siblings being affected. The figure is slightly higher, at around 10 to 15 per cent, for diagnoses of language and social skills problems that fall outside the autism spectrum. There is a higher recurrence risk of about 35 per cent when two or more siblings have ASD.

More recently, figures of up to 1 in 5 younger siblings of a child with autism being diagnosed with autism have been given. This means that the majority of siblings won't be diagnosed with autism! Most parents that I see are prepared to take this chance. They feel confident to detect early signs of autism in siblings and empowered to access timely intervention.

A genetic opinion is best reserved when you have a child with autism and known genetic condition or your child has dysmorphic (subtle, abnormal) facial features.

What do we know about autism?

This question should be: 'What don't we know about autism?' Extensive global research and networking on autism is ongoing but we still know very little about autism.

Research states that immunisations, including the MMR (measles, mumps and rubella) vaccination, do not cause autism. Neither does a 'leaky gut' or mercury (thimerosal), one of the preservatives used in some vaccines.

We do know that brain structure can be different in children with autism. Susan Greenfield, a British scientist, tells us that in the first two years of a child's life, their brain is growing exponentially. It is making multiple connections, called synapses, between individual brain cells. These synapses then connect to the various working parts of the brain and develop further as a child heads towards early adolescence.

The growing brain has much plasticity or capacity to change and remould, a term described as neuroplasticity. Yet, after having completed all that hard work, the brain prunes or discards about half of its connections, relying on and using those already assigned a role.

In autism, there is thought to be insufficient pruning. Redundant pathways somehow alter the way the brain regulates emotions, language and communication. The brain is said to be different structurally in children with autism at different stages of development, especially in the first three years when it grows too fast.

Genes in autism

We are learning that genetics has a major role in the aetiology of autism, together with modifying and external factors such as inflammation, infection and toxins. They are implicated but not yet proven.

There are more than 500 genetic mutations associated with autism and a number of close genetic syndrome linkages. These include Fragile X syndrome (FXS), Tuberous Sclerosis, schizophrenia, ADHD and mood disorders.

Fragile X syndrome

FXS is the most recognised cause for both intellectual disability and single gene cause of autism. About 5 per cent of children with autism have FXS. Autism and FXS are both more common in boys than girls.

FXS is due to a mutation (alteration) in the FMR1 (Fragile X mental retardation 1) human gene. FMR1 is important for normal brain development and female reproduction function. When this gene is changed it can't do the job it was programmed to do.

A defective gene can be passed down by a carrier parent, from a mother or father. FXS affects 1 in 3,600 males and 1 in 4,000–6,000 females. Anxiety and ADHD are also more common in children with either the pre-mutation or the full expression of this gene.

Autism comorbidity
Children with autism often have a family history of ADHD, dyslexia, dysgraphia, sensory problems, seizures, coeliac disease markers and intellectual giftedness. Family members often have problems due to anxiety, depression, tics, obsessive-compulsive symptoms, bipolar disorder and schizophrenia.

There is an overlap between the clinical presentation of autism and inattentive ADHD with language, literacy, social, anxiety and sensory problems. Perhaps some of the high functioning autism and inattentive ADHD we see as paediatricians are part of the same complex spectrum. It would help to know more about genetically linked disorders such as FXS, Tuberous Sclerosis, Tourette syndrome, ADHD, anxiety, major depression and schizophrenia.

We should consider other possible modifying factors, including toxins and pollutants in our food chain and environment. More children are presenting with allergies and autoimmune diseases such as diabetes. Adult dementia is increasing. Why is this so? When we have some answers we will know a lot more about autism.

What happens if my child has autism?
Autism awareness, acceptance, intervention and outcomes have improved. We try to diagnose children accurately and as quickly as possible. This facilitates access to appropriate, timely and

life-changing interventions and government funding before and upon entry to school.

Once a diagnosis of autism is made and recognised under a state's disability scheme, families can access financial assistance from state and federal sources to procure early autism intervention services from recognised service providers. This is a complex and changing bureaucratic process, further complicated by Australia's transition to the NDIS.

An autism advisor from your state's autism association can help you develop an appropriate financial and therapy plan to meet the specific needs of your child.

Intervention

Therapies vary and include ABA (Applied Behaviour Analysis) and Floortime. Structured speech, behavioural and sensory programs are provided by speech pathologists, clinical psychologists and occupational therapists registered to work in the area of autism.

Carol Gray's Social Stories is a widely used communication format. Thought bubbles are used to explain a social context, perspective or to illustrate social cues. Speech pathologists introduced Makaton, a communication mode which uses signs, symbols and gestures to indicate needs.

Children who have little language need some form of picture communication or electronic prompt to engage them. The Picture Exchange Communication System (PECS) uses picture cards to depict desired items or activities.

Choose and continue the treatment that best suits your child. It must start early and be best practice, consistent and intensive.

Support

Healthcare plans provide financial assistance. They are available from your local doctor, paediatrician or child psychiatrist. These are accessed under Medicare. Extra educational assistance is provided for children diagnosed with autism.

Most children with autism have their needs met in a mainstream classroom with education assistance. Some children with HFA cope very well if placed in a school environment that best suits their social, emotional and academic needs.

There are some children who have severe autism with minimal or no language. They have other conditions such as ADHD, epilepsy, genetic complexity, intellectual disability, anxiety and depression. Children with complex and debilitating problems feel frightened and distressed in a mainstream class. These children and their families deserve flexible education choices to better support their complex needs.

Management

Families and schools provide the overly sensory child with a calm and structured setting. Routine, such as regular and balanced meals and a sensible sleep pattern, provides a safety net for the fearful child. Music soothes the agitated child. Antioxidants such as omega-3 fatty acids found in fish oil may play a role in brain inflammation. Probiotics and some antibiotics may help.

Phenytoin is a medication used to treat epilepsy. Isolated case studies report that in low doses it improves the social and behavioural impairments of autism. It is not an officially recognised or approved treatment. Multivitamins, such as zinc, iron, folate, magnesium and vitamin D, and broccoli, kale and legumes could be of benefit.

Giving very low doses of a selective serotonin reuptake inhibitor (SSRI) medication boosts serotonin levels in the very anxious child. Therapists can then work optimally with them.

Keep the focus on your child. They are the same child the day of their diagnosis as they were the previous day. Your child has autism. But they still have the needs of any child. Ensure you don't lose your own identity or that of your partner and other children.

Couples sometimes split up because of the enormous emotional workload and financial devastation that follows a diagnosis of autism. Families shouldn't sacrifice their relationship, family home and other children in pursuit of a cure that is not yet available. Do what you can as a parent, but have physical, emotional and financial limit settings. Fail to implement boundaries and you may lose your family. Plan some autism-free dates in your autism treatment schedule.

Many resilient families juggle the extra demands of having a child with autism and preserve their family integrity. You can do this too. If your child is diagnosed with autism, see this as a positive diagnosis that will help you gain the necessary support to raise your child and address their unique needs.

Children with autism have many strengths. They are logical, direct and honest. This separates them from the intrigue and pettiness of social competitiveness. Celebrate every milestone that your child reaches and enjoy the journey with them.

There are 'many autisms'. I discuss how they present in each developmental stage of childhood. Further resources and references are detailed under the 'Helpful reading' part of this book.

ASD – 0 to 5 years

Language and social milestones

Knowing when it is normal for a child to smile, laugh, clap, respond and talk gives you the confidence to seek medical advice when your child is not achieving these milestones.

Most children smile by 6 to 8 weeks, babble by 5 to 6 months, respond when called by 7 months and have two to three words by 12 months. 'Dad', 'mum' and 'bub' are heard from 6 to 9 months. Some children with autism say unusual first words such as 'helicopter' and 'car'. So do 'normal' children. Language acquisition is variable in the first two years. The child who plays imaginatively during this time but is not talking may be normal. They can start speaking in sentences when they turn 3.

Twenty words by 20 months and thirty to fifty words by 2 years of age is reassuring. You need around this number to put two words together. Some 2 year olds will have up to two hundred words and already be speaking in sentences.

From the age of 2 to 3 years a child will be rapidly increasing their vocabulary. By 3 to 4 years of age, children can tell a short story using sentences of four to five words. By 4 years they have enough language experience to lie.

If your child has normal hearing but is not communicating in the first twelve months with looks, gestures, sounds or words, consider autism.

Seek professional advice if they have no single words by the age of 16 months, are not putting two words together by 2 years, or only 'talking' by repeating certain words or phrases. Children with autism repeat whole phrases of dialogue they have heard from a song or movie but are unable to engage in social conversation.

Families with autism often recall how their child appeared to be developing normally until 12, 15 or 20 months. Parents then observe their child's development to stagnate or regress. They state that their child stopped saying learned words and that their smiling, responsive child had become distant and emotionally cold.

Children who have nonverbal autism have severe deficits in their ability to speak and communicate. This is picked up earlier than the child who has normal or mildly delayed speech development. Autism may be a teenage or adult diagnosis.

Early signs of autism

A child with autism can be unsettled and irritable during infancy. So can normal babies! They may have severe colic, don't sleep or feed well, have minimal babble and poor eye contact. As a toddler they adopt a flat facial expression or avoid the gaze of strangers. They recoil when picked up or dislike handling, baths and nappy changes. Loud noises, such as the vacuum cleaner, unsettle them.

Children with autism often have extreme and persistent emotional dysregulation – they can't control their feelings. They have major temper tantrums, severe separation anxiety, mood swings, aggression and early oppositional behaviours. Parents make frequent visits to the child health nurse, chiropractor and local doctor seeking support. They attend parenting classes and trial elimination diets, fish oil, probiotics and vitamin supplements.

Babies and children who have experienced developmental trauma because of domestic violence can present with social, sensory, language and behavioural problems similar to autism. Severe postnatal depression can similarly affect the bonding and social and emotional development of the young child. When depression is detected and supported early these children demonstrate rapid improvements in social reciprocity, engagement and language. Very anxious children with significant language delay can also present with emotionally dysregulated behaviours.

Nonverbal markers of autism

Using your index finger to point to something of interest (protodeclarative pointing) is a good milestone to have. It is not always seen in autism, nor is the act of sharing and engaging in reciprocal early play or reading activities, known as 'joint attention'. Failure to develop speech, nonverbal gesturing, and protodeclarative pointing and joint attention in the first two years of life increases the likelihood of your child having autism.

Children with speech delay due to a language disorder, in contrast to autism, will still be good communicators. They look at you when they want something or show you an object. They will gesture, point and try to vocalise their needs.

Children express their developing language in early symbolic and creative play. They will model what you do and pretend to cook, clean, mow the lawn or talk on the phone. These children are unlikely to have autism, even though they are not speaking much. Play is a child's internal language. If they can't play, talk or communicate, they may have autism.

Behavioural traits

Repetitive behaviours associated with autism include lining up objects such as toy cars, trains, books, DVDs or blocks.

'Normal' children go through a stage of lining or stacking up objects, usually around the age of 2 years. Children with autism persist with these ritualistic and stereotypic behaviours.

Some children with autism will open and close doors repeatedly or look at lights for long periods. They might fixate on moving objects such as fans or water and focus on car brands, letters, colours, numbers or time. They will repetitively watch particular movies or TV shows. Children with autism relate intensely and obsessively to animated characters such as Thomas the Tank Engine, Bob the Builder, the stars of *Toy Story*, *Cars*, *Pokémon* and *Minecraft*. They are fascinated by superheroes. Some children with autism will dress only as Batman or Spiderman. 'Normal' children do these things too!

Pedantic, obsessive and repetitive behaviours with rigidity and sameness are seen in children with autism. Change is very difficult for them. A child will know the exact traffic route their parent takes to drop off older siblings at school. A change of this routine upsets them.

Young children with autism clock watch. They are driven by time and routine. These kids struggle with sudden plan changes. It is important to try to introduce some flexibility slowly into their daily routine.

Sensory signs

Children with autism are sensory seeking and sensory defensive. They dislike being touched, having their hair brushed or teeth cleaned. They place their hands over their ears when hearing loud sounds. These children get upset by the feel of clothes labels, tags and certain fabrics. The sound of fingers rubbing over synthetic or woollen fabrics disturbs them. Children will sniff objects such as books and puzzle pieces.

They are selective with their diet, have minimal iron intake and refuse to have lunch at school. Some children will only eat food that is white in colour, such as rice, fish and potato. Other children will only eat hard or crunchy foods or certain brands of cereal or yoghurt. They will refuse wet or soft foods. Forcing these kids to eat results in panic attacks or food phobia.

High pain thresholds are described in children with autism. This makes it difficult to diagnose ear, nose and throat and dental infections. It is also hard to examine a child with autism because of their anxiety and dislike of tactile contact.

Children with autism walk on their toes a lot or flap their hands when excited, afraid and anxious. They might spin and twirl. Of all these clinical signs, tiptoe walking and hand flapping are the least specific to autism. 'Normal' and anxious children do this too. Persistent and frequent spinning, rocking and head banging are more specific to autism.

Children with intellectual disabilities employ sensory-seeking behaviours. They rock their bodies, head bang or masturbate. 'Normal' children briefly go through these same phases in early childhood.

Sometimes 'normal' children, anxious children and those with a language delay will demonstrate heightened sensory and repetitive, obsessive behaviours. The difference is that in autism, these traits are pervasive, persistent and problematic throughout childhood.

ASD – 5 to 10 years

Living in the shadow of childhood

Autism is visible, symptomatic, increasing and part of the complexity of classrooms today. Children with autism find the school environment visually and socially overwhelming. An early diagnosis of autism is the best way to ensure they start school with adequate and appropriate supports in place.

All primary school classes should be 'autism friendly' and ideally funded for two teachers per class for the early educational years. Education needs to provide flexible choices for families with autism. Classrooms need to be a sensory haven for all students, conducive to promoting social and emotional resilience and a positive learning environment.

If you don't have a child with autism it is difficult to understand the subtle but definite hardship they face during their schooling.

High functioning autism
Parents and teachers struggle to comprehend the school difficulties experienced by the bright child with high functioning autism.

I have met children who have written down thousands of words so that they can learn their meaning. This is exhausting for them. They struggle with inferential language and semantic and pragmatic language (the use of language in a social context). The nuances, subtleties and humour of speech and language can be confusing for them.

Conversely, the child with high functioning autism can have strengths with verbal comprehension and vocabulary and a quirky sense of humour. They can be very creative with their writing, although with a repetitiveness and 'oddness' in their wording.

Girls with Asperger syndrome will try to emulate the different mannerisms of their socially competent peers by intense watching and mimicry. They practise facial gestures in front of a mirror for hours.

Children with HFA don't like school much. The playground can be hell for them. They feel the pain of being ostracised by peers and parents.

In class, help is limited because their disability is 'hidden'. Parents, doctors, teachers and peers will question whether the child with high functioning autism really needs the additional education assistance allocated to them.

Some children require extra assistance in the classroom. But, they already feel different and prefer to be treated the same as their peers. If they have cognitive strengths, they often cope academically. With teachers and classmates who 'get' them, they succeed at school.

Because of their sensory problems, children with autism get easily overwhelmed. They depend on the structure within their classroom to help control their emotions. Loss of routine occurs when a teacher is away, a new student arrives or when classroom furniture changes. This can cause children with HFA to display explosive and emotionally labile behaviours. They bite, hit and shove other students, sometimes with good cause.

These children are labelled 'naughty', 'difficult' or 'autistic'. What they should be called is Sebastian, Austin or Bianca!

Sensory backpacks, 'huff and puff catchers' and purple dots

A sensory classroom is a simple, uncluttered visual space with defined areas to think, read, talk, write and compute. Pre-primary and early primary school classrooms have too much visual and physical clutter. This creates anxiety in the child who needs some quiet, routine and structure. Sensory, friendly spaces should have an area for emotional debriefing or respite. A 'calm down' space. This can be a beanbag, eggchair or hammock. Earphones, music devices and supervised access to electronic screens such as iPads help some children lower their anxiety. Access to 'fidget toys' such as stress balls can help. Spinning fidget toys that contain metal are heavy and may inflict an injury if thrown, so are best kept out of classrooms.

Children can design and paint a windsock, a 'huff and puff catcher' to blow their angry thoughts into. They can make a 'worry post box' from a shoebox which they can decorate. They can post notes and pictures about their concerns.

Parents can make a sensory backpack, case or bag for their child to bring during the first week of full-time school. A suitcase with items such as bubble plastic which they can pop will help a child with autism self-soothe when upset. Place sensory shelves or lockers at the front of the classroom. The teacher grants access to these when a child needs a respite moment.

Parents know best what works for their child. A sensory backpack may not work for a child with extremely strong fixations. These children willonly go to school if they are allowed to take an object of their choosing. Other children respond to being given a range of choices, such as a Rubik's cube, Lego, a chewy necklace, plastic paperclip, favourite book, or pencils and notepad. Colouring in can be relaxing for anxious children.

Other children within the classroom learn to respect the contents and privacy of each child's sensory pack, reinforcing the importance of values of trust, honesty and integrity. A visual schedule placed on each child's desk prompts the timing of activities for each day. Parents could have a parallel visual schedule at home.

All children, not just those with autism, benefit from a visual planner. It helps relieve the anxiety of unexpected scheduling. Children like to have some control of their own lives from a young age.

For sensory children, including those with autism, a 'purple dot system' can work well. A simple purple dot is stuck onto the home or school visual schedule or diary when something happens at the last moment. This may be a change of doctor's appointment. The child with autism plans for days to see the doctor at 1 pm on a Tuesday, for example. If this time is changed, a purple dot gives them some warning that they need to cope with that change. A parent says, 'Oh look, it's a purple dot day. Let's see what is different today'.

Obsessions and repetitions

Obsessive and repetitive behaviours are seen in autism and with anxiety disorders. Fixation about time is common. Parents have to give the time in the same format. They can say, for example, 'It's six forty-five', but not 'It's a quarter to seven'. Children with autism draw multiple clock faces or fill pages with clock hands and lines of numbers. They draw dinosaurs, rabbits, cars, Lego or *Pokémon* characters. 'Normal' children will too!

'Electronic addiction' is often problematic for children with autism. Electronic screen time is used as a reward incentive for children with autism. It works well for limited periods and can be relaxing for them. *Minecraft* and Lego Star Wars games are very popular, but need to be monitored, as children can become 'addicted' to them.

Children with autism have strong visuospatial skills. They excel at electronic games. This focus can be used to encourage children with autism to develop a mutual interest in video games with like-minded peers. This provides social connectivity which would otherwise elude them.

The Secret Agent Society program is an innovative and evidence-based social skills tool which incorporates a number of computer-based games to engage and teach children with social and emotional difficulties. It is ideally suited for 8- to 12-year-old children with autism. Further details of this program are available online.

Judicious use of educational and fun apps on electronic devices including iPads can be relaxing for children with autism.

Resources and references relating to autism are provided under 'Helpful reading'.

ASD – 10 to 15 years

The 'A' in autism is for anxiety

Autism is symptomatic in the high school years because of social and performance anxiety. This is when anxiety unmasks autism that has not previously been considered or diagnosed.

Girls with high functioning autism, more commonly equated with Asperger syndrome, are the most vulnerable group. They are socially immature and present late, with high anxiety levels around Years 9 or 10, when they are 14 and 15 years of age.

Bright students with HFA can mask anxiety from teachers, doctors and even their family. This delays their diagnosis with autism until the adolescent years. They expend large amounts of mental energy learning scenarios of how to react in different situations.

High functioning autism / Asperger

Teenage girls with Asperger presentation are very good at niche hobbies such as horse dressage. They may excel in photography. They use the camera lens to see detail not appreciated by others. They may be good at music, drama and graphics or fit into the world of technology.

During the early primary school years their interests are shared with peers. They relate to electronic games such as *Minecraft, Mario,*

Simms and *Club Penguin*. They talk about characters from the movies *Star Wars, Toy Story, Cars* and *Frozen*.

When children with high functioning autism start high school the social expectations and conversation change. They feel different compared with their peers or lack this insight.

Pubertal change occurs during these transitional years. It is important for the parents of children with autism to teach them about hygiene and dress code. When I talk to teenage boys with high functioning autism, I say to them, 'The social rule is that every day you shower, use deodorant and change your socks and jocks'.

The mother of a teenage daughter with HFA told me that she forgot to provide her child with the social cue about dress code before a semi-formal event. She just presumed that her teenager would know what to wear. Her daughter attended the event but was upset that she had worn shorts and a tee-shirt. She chastised her mother for not informing her of the correct attire.

Labels

I used to think that a label of autism in the child with mild HFA or Asperger wasn't helpful. I was wrong! Colleagues and families were likewise reluctant to identify a child as being different. I had concerns about the privacy of a child and the potential for an ASD diagnosis on electronic health records and central databases, including Medicare, to impact on future vocational opportunities or insurance applications.

But, when the social struggles of a child are impacting on their emotional health and affecting them academically it is better to have a diagnosis. Teenagers say they feel different or have trouble understanding social rules such as dress code, hygiene and make-up. It's important that these kids know we are listening and that parents, psychologists and teachers are prepared to help. School becomes a more positive environment for them once people understand them better.

Schools are better funded and relieved to be given permission to help when a medical diagnosis of autism is made. This diagnostic label can be valuable for an emotionally, socially and academically struggling student. It can facilitate additional financial support. This assists families to access allied healthcare resources.

During high school, the priority is for clinical psychology and adolescent psychiatry input. This can facilitate the school applying for special consideration for the student with autism. Medication to treat anxiety or ADHD can be a helpful adjunct to therapy.

Co-education versus single gender

I think that girls with autism do better socially in a co-educational environment and in a school with a strong focus on holistic education. They embrace male humour and logic, but are confused by the social messages of teenage girls.

High academic expectation can be destructive to bright children with high functioning autism. Girls with HFA can still do well in a caring and supportive all girls' school setting. It is dependent on the child and the peer group they find at school.

Many single-stream schools with records of academic excellence recognise the risk of anxiety and perfectionism in their students. These schools are now addressing the importance of instilling emotional resilience in their primary school years. They are promoting the value of childhood play and building outdoor playgrounds to encourage children to connect with nature and each other. Some are considering the banning of homework in the early school years. I agree with their approach.

Social media

Electronic misuse can adversely influence a child's development. However, it can have a valuable role if properly managed. It provides a social lifeline for children with high functioning autism who struggle with friendships and peer acceptance. Electronic social media and electronic gaming clubs keep these kids socially connected and help them stay engaged with learning.

Problematic electronic gaming and screen use, sometimes referred to as an 'addiction' is uncommon in children with a normal developmental trajectory. But, it occurs more frequently in children and adolescents with a major depressive or other mental health problem.

Part 5

Childhood from 5 to 10

Ever tried. Ever failed.
No matter. Try again.
Fail again. Fail better.

Samuel Beckett

The gift of childhood

Hold onto childhood

'Can a child remember being five years of age?' 'Yes'. 'Are child-hood memories important?' 'They are to the child'. Significant milestones of these childhood years are emotional and social resilience, language and learning. They have a pivotal role in this stage of childhood growth and development.

This is the time when a child's anxiety, social awkwardness, learning difficulties and family conflict can carve a defining path in their journey.

Childhood memories

'Children's footsteps aren't made in the sand; they are made in cement and last forever' – Kim Oates, paediatrician.

Childhood memories start between 3 and 4 years of age, or possibly earlier if stimulated by a highly emotive event. The prior period of 'childhood amnesia' is like a child being backstage. When it's their time, the child enters the stage and becomes part of the act.

Living in an emotionally intense moment cements memories, both good and bad. That is why some vulnerable children struggle to free themselves from the grip of childhood adversity. Some of these memories are transgenerational and remain powerful and influential over time.

A grandfather, close to 80 years of age, spoke little about his childhood. One day he disclosed that a significant adult figure in his childhood would nag him for hours. He was forced to sit still on a kitchen stool and listen to a relentless barrage of cruel words.

I then understood his need for solitude. Early childhood memories define our future selves. The emotion of early childhood can distort a child's memory. A bad memory can displace those which would otherwise have been good.

We need to give our children pleasant-tasting and wonderful-smelling memories.

The art of praise

Too much applause

To instil emotional resilience back into childhood, we have to stop overpraising children. Not everything a child does is a 'good job'. If they don't learn this, they can't develop strategies to tackle challenges as they grow.

Kids need to see that adults don't always get it right. They need to see mum or dad fail, or their teacher misspell a word.

Many schools have got rid of stickers and gold stars. Ribbons for swimming and running races are awarded to place getters alone. Children understand this. They don't value a ribbon for coming sixth.

Coming home from work one day, I was driving behind a large family car. Plastered on the rear window was their child's sporting award from a local Australian junior football club. It said 'Class Act Award' and 'Best Team Player'.

This doesn't send a good message to that child. How can they do better or achieve more? This type of 'overpraise' has the potential to set them up for failure and to incite sibling or peer rivalry.

Parents and teachers find it hard to change behavioural approaches that have become so ingrained. Getting the balance right between positively or negatively encouraging a child can be tricky. How much praise is enough? It's a bit like asking, 'How much is a pinch of salt?'

I once witnessed an exchange between a junior school principal and a Year 2 student. The small child had written a story and was keen to share it with a teacher. I recall the child holding up her creative manuscript of hurried scrawl, her face beaming above the crumpled page. The teacher held the story in her hands and then returned it to the child. She told the child to write more neatly next time. I saw that child's exuberance and passion die in the middle of a concrete playground. It was a long time before that little girl wrote again.

Teachers grasp the hearts of young children. It is an awesome responsibility. There is a balance between overpraise and criticism. It is called positive acknowledgement.

I have often thought about those few words spoken by a very experienced and caring teacher. How could she have said them better?

If you are a teacher or parent reading this, reflect and think about what you will say when a child shares their masterpiece. Avoid stating that a child's work is the best you have ever seen. They will feel they can't reproduce such excellence again.

The teacher could have said, 'I like the way you have described the characters in your story and I am looking forward to how you are going to write about them in your next one'.

Childhood SPECS – 5 to 10 years

Language

Children should now have mastered receptive and expressive language skills. They can listen, comprehend, converse and manipulate language. A child of 9 can hear and understand most adult conversation but won't have developed inferential and more complex language concepts. They struggle to interpret language.

In middle childhood the brain is still doing lots of networking and forming neural connections. This is when parents should encourage their children to read and improve their vocabulary. It is not the time for 'lazy learning' from tablets or iPads to be prioritised.

Physical development

The primary school years are when kids grow their muscles. To do this they need time to exercise and get physically fit. They can't do this by sitting in front of an electronic screen for hours each day.

In the past, even very young children walked or rode a bike to school. This ritual has been replaced with the drive-through pick-up or 'kiss and drop' zones. Children don't get enough exercise. They have poorly defined calf muscles.

Children have limited outdoor exposure to sunlight. They wear hats and sunscreen and select sedentary activities. They have low vitamin D levels, especially in winter because of lack of sunlight.

Healthy lunches are supplemented by too many snacks. Lack of exercise and excess calories contribute to childhood obesity.

Some children lose weight. Children on medication for the treatment of ADHD can have appetite suppression and eat too little. Children with certain medical conditions such as cystic fibrosis have to eat high-fat diets to maintain their weight.

Childhood obesity

If you look back over old family photographs, people appear thin. Calories have impregnated our staple foods by stealth. Meal sizes are larger. Children eat more and exercise less. This leads to obesity. In later life, bone loss (osteoporosis) and sugar imbalance occurs. Children who are grossly overweight get early onset type 2 diabetes. This was once an old person's disease.

Inactivity is a simple lifestyle issue which every parent has the power to change. We need to raise healthier children who exercise more, connect with nature and spend fewer hours in front of screens. This makes more sense than introducing a tax on high sugar–content drinks and will have a positive effect on childhood behaviour. Regular exercise is protective for the physical and mental health of young children.

Social and emotional development

Extracurricular activities are the best way of engaging kids with interests, challenges and connecting them with their peer group. They help separate study and play. Assign your child a winter and a summer sport each year. Offer a choice of two. This gives them ownership of their decision. Don't provide too many options.

If the family budget permits, consider a musical instrument, drama, dance or art. Participation in Scouts or Cadets can provide social connectivity, enhance social awareness and promote leadership skills. Teach your child a second language.

Children's joints and voices can be damaged from early and inappropriate overuse. This can occur if children have formal singing lessons too early or spend excessive hours physically training. Elite sporting and dance programs require parental surveillance to ensure your child retains adequate life balance. Children must have sufficient time to develop peer friendships and socialise during their early growing years. This makes them happy.

If your child demonstrates early musicality, explore ways to develop this that will foster their love of music. Not every child who plays the violin or piano will become a concert performer. Ensure it is your child who wants to pursue music excellence and not yourself.

Your child doesn't have to be good at music, sport or art to enjoy these activities. They just need to have a go. The child who disengages from all extracurricular activities will have limited opportunity to build strong emotional and social resilience.

Cognitive growth and learning

Academic demands increase exponentially through the early school years. Your child will cope if they have strong emotional and social resilience. This is a better predictor of school success than an IQ score.

Children think, reason and conceptualise more as they move from pre-primary to Year 5.

A 6-year-old boy was asked what he would want if granted three wishes. He looked at me quizzically, but couldn't think of anything. This is quite common in children of this age. They can be shy or perhaps they already have everything they need. Other young children will ask for more money, lots of 'candy', computer games or Lego. His older brother when asked the same question enquired whether it was about friends or things.

Childhood feelings

Children need friends

Friendships are important during the formative years of primary school. Year 3 is a difficult social year. It is the time when class birthday invites stop. As a parent you share your child's disappointment when coloured envelopes containing fancy invitations bypass them. Birthdays are best organised outside school boundaries to minimise social exclusion. You also need to teach your child that not everybody can be included on the party list.

Friendships are created and cliques evolve during these early years. Children learn about bullying, how to be a friend and how to cope with losing friends. Schools often organise social skills training courses for children in Year 2, 3 or 4. These are run by speech pathologists or clinical psychologists.

Drama groups are a good way of teaching social skills in a creative, fun and safe environment. Books provide safe social stories and strategies about growing up.

Starting school is like going to the beach for the first time. Would you rush into the water with your child before looking to see if there were any rips or unsafe areas? School is the same. Meet and greet new peers and their parents but avoid rushing into play dates too enthusiastically. When you accept or offer that first play date, make it at your home for two or four children. Limit the duration of the play or agree to meet at a local children's playground. Good friendships are often founded on mutual ground.

Ready for school?

Early childhood education

Busy has become an excuse for failing to teach our children to read in the early school years. The primary school curriculum is cluttered with too many subjects and teaching methods. If educators are confused about how to teach literacy, no wonder parents, grandparents and children struggle. Keep learning simple, fun and structured.

I favour a holistic approach to education and provision for extending the intellectually gifted child within that framework whilst prioritising the social and emotional development of the child. I have concerns about a national curriculum which, if too rigid, limits the ability of discerning teachers to teach outside narrow education parameters. This leads to a low expectation from education.

Education should cover the core learning areas of numeracy, literacy and digital literacy (coding). Mastering the skill of coding allows students to 'talk' to computers and direct how they function. Students will struggle in a technologically advanced world if they fail to gain this competency. Financial literacy is also important for students.

Effective teachers have to be competent in at least one of these areas, and for primary school teaching in all of them. Teaching directives should not discriminate against visual learners who require an avenue for oral presentation in order to shine. Most of all, an early childhood school curriculum must not lose sight of providing children with the language skills to communicate with each other.

Schools are burdened with the responsibility of teaching social values of respect, kindness and social justice. Not all children are learning these life skills at home.

Education is about inciting passion in a student to learn so they can convert information into knowledge. It is about the student and teacher 'fit', not about manipulating grades and tweaking league table results.

Most importantly, education should give children a sense of belonging. This makes them feel valued and worthwhile. They will be less likely to seek cult or gang acceptance later.

Literacy

There are moves to simplify the primary school curriculum and teach children how to read by direct instruction and the use of phonics.

Phonics is the study of phonemes which are the basic distinctive units of speech sound. After being exiled from the classroom, phonics is back. It is prominent in children's books written by innovative authors such as Dr Seuss, Mem Fox, Pamela Allen and Eric Carle.

Some schools teach early reading skills by a chance approach. They get kids to look at the vibe of the word and work it out. This is called learning by the 'whole language' method. The move to shift our education focus and reintroduce phonics to the school curriculum is good. It will help children read.

Reading is like music. On some musical instruments you learn individual notes, then chords and finally songs. Once kids understand individual and groups of sounds they can start to read words, then sentences. As they practise these steps, reading becomes more fluent. Good parents and teachers know when and how to push this process along so that children end up reading fluently.

Visual readers

Intellectually gifted children often teach themselves how to read. They are reading by 3 to 4 years. Bright children can also have early reading lag and avoid choosing a book at school. This is often missed in the visual learner. They fudge their way through the first year or two of school by remembering words through picture linkage.

If you are reading with your child, try covering the picture briefly. See if your child understands the words. If they can't read them, discuss this with your teacher. Your child may benefit from a language and learning assessment with a speech pathologist or a developmental and educational psychologist. Teachers will be supportive of their input. The teacher is on your side and wants your child to learn.

Most children need adult help to read. They don't read until they are 5 or 6 years of age. This is normal. Some schools and education systems favour a focus on play and defer formal reading instruction until a child is close to 7 years old.

Dyslexie font

Children with dyslexia require lots of support, patience, encouragement and flexible teaching methods. Dyslexie is a specific font that appears easier for children with dyslexia to read. A number of popular books are to be printed using this typeface.

Alongside reading

Praise and reward won't instil the love of reading in the reluctant student. Kids might read when coerced, but won't embrace books. It is better for the child to choose a story they love, make a habit of alongside reading each day and read for fun.

Your job as a parent is to provide a rich pre-literacy home environment for your young child. Children must be developmentally ready to read and have consolidated their pre-literacy skills before being forced to read at school. Otherwise, they will develop a fear or phobia about words and reading and fail.

If your child is always picking easy books they could lack confidence with their reading skills. As well as 10 minutes of reading with your child every day, reading an instructional book which utilises phonics and visual prompts can be valuable. A classic text for children from 5 to 9 years is *Teach Your Child to Read in 100 Easy Lessons* by Siegfried Engelmann. This is available online and at bookstores.

Intellectual giftedness

You may have a child who is reading and problem-solving before they enter the school system, who asks lots of questions and has a strong sense of social justice. Prepare for the challenge of raising a gifted child. It can be extremely difficult.

Intellectually gifted children often have advanced early literacy skills. They feel disconnected from their peers and frustrated with a curriculum that is age, and not stage, pitched. When their intellect is recognised they can be burdened with the extra work of extension programs. They struggle with perfectionism, identity and social fit. This is problematic for the gifted child who also has autism, anxiety or a high IQ with a specific learning disorder such as dyslexia or ADHD.

Recognising the social and emotional needs of these children is more important than praising their intellectual gifts. Visits to the zoo, library, parks and literacy, computing, drama, music, art and sport have an active role in the education of the very bright child.

Emotional and cognitive mismatch

Leta Hollingworth, an early American psychologist and pioneer of intellectual giftedness, was credited as saying, 'It is difficult to have the intelligence of an adult and the emotions of a child in a childish body'.

A Year 2 primary school student discovered that if she acted poorly her name was placed outside the 'love heart' drawn on the board by her teacher. She was then sent to another classroom where she learned new and exciting stuff with a teacher that she liked. Her behaviour within the classroom she hated did not improve. She was extremely bright but had the 'disability' of an early emotional and cognitive IQ mismatch. When

*combined with a poor student–teacher fit she presented with dysregulated
and emotionally labile behaviours.*

If the mismatch of social and emotional factors persists and is a
part of the intrinsic school and peer culture, you have to consider
a different school environment. In this specific clinical case, a
dedicated, experienced senior relief teacher advised the family to
remove the child from the school and her peer group.

This can be a very difficult decision and is best made with
objective professional advice. This child was fortunate to move
to a school that better understood her language, walked in her
shoes and created a space for her. A new teacher 'got' her unique
needs. This positive change was effected by a caring teacher who
advocated for a child and prioritised the needs of the child above
the pride of a school. Such actions define the gifted educator.

Shifting schools

Parents must think carefully before changing schools. This needs
to be a rational decision, made on social and emotional grounds
and not just academic concerns. The education of a child is more
dependent on the emotional stability and happiness of the child
than their intellectual ability. Professional advice can be sought
from a paediatrician, psychiatrist or clinical psychologist. Changing
schools too late can result in a poor outcome. Parents should take
charge and make these decisions early.

Once a student has reached Year 8 or 9, any change demands
great resilience from the adolescent and a supportive school and
peer group. Most importantly, the adolescent must be on board or
it is unlikely to work. They will sabotage your parental decision
to prove a point, even if their new school is 'better'. A school must
be better for the child, not just the parents.

What do children think about?

Children think about sex

Young children are curious. They ask lots of questions. When parents get busy it is easy to dismiss or deflect them. 'Go and ask your father', 'I'll tell you later' or 'Mummy is busy, play with my phone for a bit' are not good answers. Talk with your child, especially when you are busy.

Young children ask, 'How are babies made?' or 'Where do they come from?' They just want a simple, age-appropriate answer. A 5-year-old child doesn't need to know intricate details. They might just want confirmation that there is a baby in mummy's tummy. There are great picture books and online resources to assist parents to answer their children's difficult questions.

The 'facts of life'

Even when children are young it is best to be honest about the 'facts of life'. Avoid using euphemisms for body parts. A girl has a vagina and a boy has a penis. This avoids confusion. It can be helpful when discussing protective behaviours such as good and bad touching.

Young children are inquisitive and masturbate. Children with an intellectual disability do this more openly. Childhood masturbation does not equate with sexual abuse.

Sex education

I think that most parents still defer sex education to schools. Sometimes their child is not ready to discuss the mechanics of sex. Children need the correct version of sex before they get this from uninformed peers. However, it is just as important that a young child learns about sexual boundaries, kindness, appropriate hugs, affection and positive relationship. This protects them from the sexualisation of children which occurs in our media. Sexualisation is a term used to describe the focus of children's appeal being due to their physical appearance and sexual attractiveness rather than their innate characteristics.

This concept is facilitated by the 'selfie' and 'sexting'. The narcissistic digital posting and sharing of self has promoted sexiness rather than self. It has taken the relationship out of sex.

Schools are under pressure to introduce sex education into their curriculum earlier. There is talk about raising transgender concepts in primary school and same-sex marriage in pre-primary classes. Sensitive topics benefit from input with the school community and should be age and stage appropriate.

Puberty

Children commence puberty at an earlier age than their parents or grandparents. In the past, girls would start breast development, which marked the start of puberty, when they were 10 or 11 years of age. Precocious or abnormally early puberty defined sexual change prior to the age of 8 years. It is now common to see girls from 8 to 9 years of age with early breast bud development. Periods usually start around two years after breast bud development. This means that your child is likely to have her first period in primary school. In the past, girls would be closer to 13 years before their menarche.

Children as young as 3 years can appear to have breasts. Mostly this is a benign condition called premature thelarche (early breast development). It usually stagnates or regresses. If it progresses or is associated with signs of early puberty, such as pubic and axillary hair, body odour, acne and vaginal blood discharge, it requires medical management. This should be with a paediatrician or paediatric endocrinologist doctor.

Boys with early puberty will grow larger testicles and their penis will get bigger. The start of male puberty is when the testicles are 4 millilitres in volume, around the size of a grape.

Sex in the media

Children now have greater exposure to 'sex' than their parents. It is pervasive and can be both confrontational and subliminal. Advertisers know that sex sells. That's why we see so much of it on TV, magazines, YouTube, computer games and books. Children see sexualisation as normal by what people around them say, wear and do.

You might censor your home from sexually explicit material, but at some stage your child will be exposed to it at a sleepover or with friends. You can't raise your child in a media vacuum.

Children are a captive, influential and potentially lucrative audience for advertising bodies and big business. Some would say that we have lost the battle against the sexualisation of children and teenagers. It has become imprinted and too accepted in the fabric of our society. Parents have the power to shift this unhealthy pattern of child development. It is called consumerism. They can say no to sexy knickers for 5 year olds. If a product doesn't sell, it dies.

Children think about gender

Children can tell you if they are a boy or a girl from around the age of 3 years. But, there are some children who feel they are living in the wrong body. These are the transgender children who want to 'switch'.

This is an area outside my expertise and best approached with an expert based at a major children's teaching hospital in your state.

Don't judge these children or families. We don't walk in their shoes. Paediatricians look after all children.

Children think about dying

Families know with harsh reality that children as young as 6 and 7 years old think about dying. Some try to die and some succeed. This increasingly tragic trend is being perpetuated in our teenage cohort. Worryingly, more teenage girls are turning to suicide as a solution.

Suicide

Our caring community is increasingly aware of suicide. It is talked about more openly. Facing the reality of suicide helps us better manage and prevent the loss of young and purposeful lives.

As parents we must listen and talk with children. Remember to tell them that we love and value them. That we are there to help. Acknowledge a child's sadness and the perception that their life is not worthwhile. It is not useful to tell a depressed person that life is okay. It is not for them. Maybe we will get a chance to give them other options and choices. Sadly, sometimes we can't. But we always have to try. There are many professional services to help us. I have listed contact details for suicide prevention under anxiety and depression in the resource section of this book.

Support services

If you have cared or are caring for a young child who is very anxious, sad and withdrawn, seek professional help. It can be hard to get, but keep asking and searching. Help can be from the child health nurse, teacher, school nurse, counsellor or psychologist.

Contact a social worker, local doctor, paediatrician or child psychiatrist. Resort to a helpline or online resource.

Families present in crisis to their local hospital or tertiary children's hospital emergency department. They may have to call mental health crisis services or the police.

Facing death

It is best to be honest with children about death.

The tragedy of death is always unexpected and uninvited. It takes the innocence of childhood and affects us all. We hear about global tragedies now because of social media and the immediacy of the news which blasts at us 24/7. We don't have to listen to bad news. Parents can monitor the frequency and nature of the news to which their children are exposed.

> *A little girl had just turned 4 years of age. She looked through a picture book and pointed to the faces on each page. She kept saying, 'Sad'. Her father said she was worried and quiet after watching a movie in which one of the characters died. This was a popular animated movie and one watched by many children. Children can sense emotion through their skin. They breathe and feel it. Sadness and loss are important emotions for a young child to learn. We need to be cognisant of this.*

The pace of childhood

Electronic innovation and technology takeover

When I reflect on my childhood and that of my own children I see the enormity of difference in our lifestyles – the simplicity of mine, the complexity of theirs. I was raised in a house devoid of white noise. There was no television until I was 10 years of age, no videos or DVDs.

I sat in a classroom in 1969 listening on a wireless to the strained sounds of the first man to walk on the moon. Kids today access a virtual classroom and see images of Pluto downloaded by NASA on Instagram. I wonder how their children will learn. If history repeats, our society will fail to learn the lessons of ancient Rome and other great civilisations, and we may be reading from books again!

Simple treats

As a child, my three top-rated treats were rainbow-coloured greaseproof paper, packet biscuits and ice-cream on a stick. My teenage daughters hanker after brown recycled paper or newspaper to wrap gifts, homemade wholesome snacks and certified organic yoghurt. This is what I call 'the circle of life'.

Play

My children are now emerging adults. Their fondest childhood memories are those of fun and simplicity, engaging in make-believe play at the beach, playing shops in their cubby and listening to stories. They are not about flying to Europe or seeing great plays. Although, sitting centre stage in the dress circle in the West End in London, watching Nick Jonas in *Les Miserables* was well received!

We are now paying people to teach young children to play. Events which get kids outdoors, being active and creative are over-subscribed. Families see the value of making kites, constructing cubbies from cardboard boxes and enjoying the company of other children.

Parents spend money on buying special sand for their children that doesn't make a mess. Why not just go outside and play in normal sand? Simple play is a great way of instilling social rules and values and promoting leadership. Families need to put aside time to engage and play regularly with their young children. The 10-year-old child is not too old to play. Neither is your 16 year old. Children just want time with their parents!

Electronic babysitters

The Millennial Generation or Generation Y – children born from the early 1980s to the 2000s – captures my parenting experience. Parents of this era were too quick to embrace the electronic revolution. We became complacent and lazy with our parenting.

My children had exposure to electronic babysitters. They had access to TV, DVDs, videos, radios, iPods, iPads, smartphones, tablets, computers, PlayStation, Wii and electronic games. They could communicate by electronic sign language, using text, MSN, Skype and email.

The experts tell us that children can't have email accounts and that they shouldn't have access to social media and age-restricted sites such as Kik and Facebook. Yet some children under 10 years are active on social media. Very young children hop onto YouTube or surf the internet without their parents' knowledge. Many parents fail to keep abreast with technology. Parents have to keep up with our digital world to effectively parent today's kids. Technology is part of life. We all have to learn to use it and not be afraid.

There are helpful online sites to guide you about the risks of young children having inappropriate access to the internet and walk you through cybersafety rules. I have included some of these in the resource section.

Screen eyes

Screen time can steal childhood

Problematic internet use due to excessive computer and internet engagement can lead to electronic addiction, emotional distress and functional impairment.

Children of all ages and particularly boys can become 'addicted' to online electronic gaming sites. It is a risk when children have access to unlimited and unsupervised screen time.

This is a parenting problem. We have to learn how to parent in the real and digital world. Failure to navigate an electronic world can cause problematic internet use and electronic addiction. This could have a public health impact on our homes, schools and workplaces and affect our children's mental health.

Electronic media gives us the benefits of innovative technology. Injudicious use brings us the consequences of altered social and emotional connectivity, and the invasion of privacy and theft of our time.

Electronic media can steal the imagination and time of a child. If children are not given sufficient time to play, they limit their ability to develop internal language, self-talk, problem-solve and think creatively. Language and peer interactions are affected.

Inappropriate use of electronic devices such as smartphones, iPads, tablets and computers can cause children to become stressed. They act out physically and emotionally if they cannot get their daily 'fix' of electronic screen time. Children become aggressive and anxious.

It can be very demanding and tiring as a parent to take control and place firm boundaries on computer time. Healthy screen time for all the family is an important parenting goal. Parents can achieve this by instilling sensible practices on the safe use of electronic screen time within the household during the early childhood years. If you fail to do this early, it is impossible to win this battle with an adolescent.

Screen time balance

Screen time is an important part of childhood. It affects the social, emotional and cognitive development of our children. The American Academy of Pediatrics (AAP) have formatted new guidelines for the healthy use of screen time in young children and adolescents. They focus on the role of parents in helping children create a balance of creative play on and off the screen. Children who spend excessive time watching screens, particularly in their bedroom 'caves', are vulnerable to developing obesity and to early sexualisation and sex predators.

Their shift in policy from previously recommending a maximum of two hours of screen time each day recognises that children have to learn how to survive in a digital world.

Healthy digital diets

A number of online sites talk about healthy electronic screen use. They include Digital Nutrition, Common Sense Media and the Australian Council on Children and the Media (ACCM).

Additional resources are found in the 'Helpful reading' section of this book.

Connecting with childhood

The value of childhood play

My children had organised play. This was dictated by nannies or the rules of paid play at Gymbus, Jungle Gym or Gymbaroo. Life was squeezed in between going to the swimming pool, tennis courts or music and drama lessons. Little time was left for them to devise their own fun.

Give your child the gift of time to think, reflect, play and do. Allow yourself equal time to meditate and absolve the busyness of your parenting life.

A parent or grandparent's greatest challenge in caring for children between the ages of 5 and 10 years is to encourage them to play without electronic and media props.

Walking along the Swan River in Perth one Saturday morning, I saw some active young children of around 5 to 6 years throwing some brightly coloured balls. This was an organised sport activity for kids and one of the emerging businesses which instruct your child on how they should play, run and have fun.

There is a trend to encroach on public spaces with expensive organised play and equipment. Simple play in open spaces is a great leveller for kids. It should remain accessible to all social and cultural groups. We shouldn't polarise our communities by demarcating parks, gardens and open spaces with paid play.

Play spaces

The physical environment created by green space and the schoolyard is important for young children. Children live in crowded housing conditions with little space to play. Some new homes look pretty but they have no grass, dirt, cubby, trees or room for adventure. Children will always opt for these basics over a pristine al fresco and barbecue area if given the choice.

Schools need open areas for kids to play. Play equipment is a great equaliser for children. It promotes socialisation and helps children learn to deal with conflict. A child does not have to compete with their peers when hanging from the monkey bars or climbing equipment. I always smile when I ask kids what games they play at recess. Primary school children still say chasey, tag or variants of this timeless game. This response restores my hope in childhood.

Kids hate being cooped up in a confined space all day. Early childhood classrooms would benefit from having a 'kid run' in a corridor alongside the classroom. Active children, especially boys and kids with hyperactive ADHD, would benefit from a run every half hour or so.

Physical exercise relieves tension, anxiety and settles the child down so that they can then better focus on their schoolwork. Brief intense periods of exercise on a daily basis or regular sustained exercise can even be therapeutic for our mental health.

Innovative thinking is reforming childhood education. Adults are starting to acknowledge the value of play and childhood imagination. There is greater recognition of the importance of tactile play. Children are given permission to touch dirt, sand and mud and to get dirty.

Sterile environments painted with bleaches and antiseptics are blamed for making children less resistant to infection and increasing childhood allergy.

The community and families want parks and open spaces. They are starting to stand up against greedy land developers. Play remains an important part of childhood.

The right to play

Children who live in isolated areas have limited opportunities to play with peers. Children who move frequently or are forced to move home, school or country lose friends. This is emotionally traumatic. It must be especially so for those children held in detention.

Caring adults need to advocate for the rights of children to play, to provide opportunities to connect with their peer group and to have safe havens in which to connect with peers, imagine and create.

Busy can spoil childhood

Busyness and electronic connectivity have restricted a child's accessibility to childhood. It has taken time away from the parent–child relationship.

Most 4-year-old girls have outgrown Barbie dolls and fairies. Boys seek visually violent movies and electronic games from a young age. As adults we should try to encourage a child to hold onto their imaginative and creative play for as long as possible. This allows them to form a strong identity of self.

The primary school years disappear quickly. This is an important time for your child's emotional, social and academic growth. It is a time for parents to be vigilant and to keep children on the parental radar. Kids watch and learn from what you say, eat, drink and smoke. They observe your attitudes and mannerisms; the way you connect to social media. They are affected by the way you treat them, yourself, your partner, friends and other people.

These middle childhood years are a time to be kind and patient. Children notice the body language of their parents. If this says, 'I don't respect your mother or your father', then children don't have a strong role model to take into their own adult lives and relationships.

Children who are raised in a household where there is tension, inconsistency, uncertainty, alcohol and drug abuse and domestic violence are especially vulnerable to mental health problems. This is why the village is so important in the raising of our children. It is why children have to be able to trust adults in a position of power. Children must be safe in the care of teachers, sports coaches, community leaders and other parents.

Be the adult

Battle of the wills

Most people don't 'see' young children. They can be noisy and annoying, drop ice-cream cones on the footpath, stick chewing gum under seats and hide behind iPads at restaurants. Children of 5 to 10 years can be feisty. They have a very loud voice. This is an age of the battle of the wills. It is important for parents to retain an adult role in robust encounters with these children.

My father was fair and consistent with his parenting. He and I had a few battles as we learned how to navigate childhood.

When I was 8 years old I needed new school sandals. My father took me to Young's General Store in Kununurra to purchase them. All the shoes were neatly arranged in pairs. I saw my shoes straight away. They were the gold and white strappy sandals on the top shelf. On the bottom shelf were the classic white fringe and buckle sandals that were practical, comfortable and affordable.

I pleaded with my father to buy the gold sparkly sandals. He stood firm in his stance to purchase sensible, durable footwear. We left the store with the standard white school shoes in a box. By the time we arrived home I had ripped the lining from them so that they couldn't be worn. But, my father had superglue and my shoes were fixed.

As soon as the glue had dried I painted them bright green with some shoe colouring I had found at the bottom of my mother's wardrobe. My reasoning was that no father would allow their child to go to school with bright green feet. I had not reckoned on the resolve of my father.

This was one battle that I lost. There are some confrontations that parents must win. These can be defining lessons in the life course of a child.

Good parenting requires tough love and parental fortitude, especially when the battle is with a young, determined child. It also needs 'Green's Law'. This states that the resilience of the adult must exceed that of the child.

This story affirms the value of calm and resolute parenting. My father earned my respect that day. There was no anger, shouting or hitting. My father was the adult and in control.

Respect children

Never disrespect the intelligence of a child or belittle their importance. Children only give a parent or teacher one chance. You need to recognise when you are being sized up by them.

I witnessed a 7 year old dismiss the credibility of a good clinical psychologist upon their first meeting. The young child was in Year 2 at school. She was short in stature but tall in discernment and opinion. The psychologist was introduced to the child but called her by an incorrect name. When asked how old she was, the child falsely stated that she was 5 years old and was in kindergarten. The psychologist had a slim chance of recovering from this situation as she failed to respond to this falsehood.

The mother recognised that a therapeutic relationship was not possible and intervened to terminate the session before it had begun. She completed the session at the local coffee shop with her child.

Believe in children

Adults need empowerment to have a go at life. So do children. Belief, trust and respect of childhood are the ways to inspire children to engage in new tasks and experience success. It is how children build up self-confidence.

An elderly man recalled a childhood with little affirmation. School was unpleasant and stressful. However, this grandfather had one happy school memory which altered his life. His teacher was absent for a day and he had to sit in another class. The new teacher asked his students, 'What was different about a moth and a butterfly?' A smile emerged from beneath his wrinkles as he recalled the response he gave as a 7-year-old child – 'A moth will fly towards the light'. The teacher affirmed his answer and a small child was given a sense of importance which he carried with him throughout life.

That teacher believed in a vulnerable child and gave him hope. Many successful adults owe their life trajectory to one teacher who made a difference.

Don't blink or you will miss childhood

A Moment in Childhood

A small child walks a path,
Shadowed by a falling leaf.

It flutters as the wind breathes,
Then stills, lying resilient and proud.

I see the stretched smile,
Full of life and hope, empty of sound.

The car engines, loud and impatient,
Racing each other at the lights.

Green light flashes, reality restored.
Glancing back, a small figure blurred.

Childhood lingers, its smell embedded,
Hovering, like the leaf.

Our daughter decided to skip being 10 and fast-track adolescence. This coincided with a parenting talk by psychologist Michael Carr-Gregg. He explained the premise that one day you wake up and in your child's bed lies the teenager you are yet to know.

That very night our daughter was busy in her room. When I popped outside to put the rubbish away, she was a little girl. Her room was adorned with Barbies, unicorns, fairy paraphernalia and soft hues of pinks, blues and purples. When I came inside, her room was lined with Michael Jackson posters. There were lots of shoeboxes stacked up in the wardrobe as coffins in which lay Bratz dolls, Barbies and the remnants of Little Pony's long flowing mane, waving goodbye to childhood.

204

I was stunned. This milestone happened just as quickly and unexpectedly as my child's first steps.

The message of this story is to ensure that you take time to embrace and enjoy your child's early years. Don't miss childhood by being too busy and important. You will wake up one day and it is gone.

Take time to enjoy every precious childhood moment. It will make you a happier and better parent.

The challenge of parenting

Armchair experts

Talkback radio is an important social platform. But, it can't exclude the grumpy people who complain about unruly kids, juvenile delinquency, the disintegration of society and failed parents. Experts can sometimes denigrate parents, judging them as over-protective and too busy hovering, rescuing, smothering or ignoring their children to parent effectively.

It is not helpful to stereotype parents and condemn them into the 'bad parent' corner. They may be just you or me, needing a tweak or a tug to shift the focus back onto our kids. Children respond to positive parenting. So do parents.

We need to be emotionally available and time-free to talk to our kids. We can't do this if we are struggling with our own physical and mental health issues or have an unrealistic workload. An elite cohort of perfect parents, grandparents or experts remain emotionally distanced from childhood. They can lack compassion and understanding of the emotionally tumultuous task of raising a child today.

It is argued that raising children in the postwar years was just as hard as today's parenting. Difficulty is about perception. Parenting today has more complex layers.

Parenting has changed

We live in a climate of social shift with new rules defined by the pervasive influence of electronic media. Conversation is no longer simple. Social connectivity ostracises those who choose to ignore technology. Failure to embrace and actively manage technology and to be familiar with electronic devices is akin to refusing to hook up your home to a landline or TV aerial in the 1970s. Electronic devices and their potential misuse are just part of the complex fabric of modern parenthood.

The childhood years from 5 to 10 are when adults need to both nurture and challenge their child. They have to be around to pick their child up when they fail. This period of growth can determine how strong a child grows, and what they can strive to do. The words tossed to a child stay with that child and can be powerful, so are best chosen carefully.

My adult dream

What type of childhood would I now choose for my children? A less busy and more private one. I am sure that this would also be their choice.

If I could live a dream it would be to restore imagination, time, simplicity, quiet and play to childhood, to value children and give them a sense of belonging. To gift children with autism the magic of language, communication and socialisation – to take anxiety out of childhood.

Part 6

More cruel friends

All about attention deficit hyperactivity disorder (ADHD)

If your child is under 5 years of age, don't read this yet, unless they are a busy, accident-prone kid and you have been asked, 'Has your child got ADHD?' This is the last diagnosis to make in a very young child. There are too many other things it could be. Your child could have a hearing problem and so can't listen. They may be intellectually gifted and overly inquisitive and demanding. Or, they are a normal busy 4-year-old child!

What is ADHD?

ADHD is a neurodevelopmental disorder. This means it affects the way the brain develops, thinks, plans, remembers and acts. It can alter the ability to reflect, self-regulate, organise, prioritise and motivate. These are our executive functioning skills. They are better determinants of social and academic success than our measured intelligence.

When we struggle with executive functioning it is hard to listen, focus, attend, concentrate and follow instructions. It is easy to procrastinate, rush tasks and not complete them. Consistency is not a strength, but when interested in a topic, great work can be produced.

ADHD is in our genes. It is often linked with a family history of specific learning problems, motor and vocal tics, anxiety, depression, bipolar disorder and schizophrenia. About 5 to 7 per cent of children and 4 per cent of adults have ADHD. Some cases of ADHD get better or become less symptomatic in adult life, whilst some adults have undiagnosed ADHD. They have problematic personal and workplace relationships.

Types of ADHD

Children with inattentive ADHD have problems listening, concentrating and managing their time and priorities. They often daydream and dawdle. They find it hard to plan, organise, initiate and write, edit and rewrite their work. They are slow to complete their work and get anxious when placed under time constraints.

These kids forget to take pencils, lunch or homework to school. They will lose a shoe, their glasses, phone or sports bag and are often disorganised and messy. Children with predominant inattentive ADHD often have language-based learning and other problems. These are called comorbidities and include anxiety, depression, tic disorder and autism.

ADHD with inattention is just one of the three forms of ADHD. The other two are ADHD with inattention and hyperactivity and

ADHD with hyperactivity and impulsivity. Most kids have the combined form. They have difficulty staying still and being focused.

Most people have heard about ADHD with hyperactivity and impulsivity. This describes the effervescent and explosive 'gas in a bottle' children. ADHD kids struggle socially. They don't always respect the personal space of others. They interrupt conversations, talk incessantly and lack a pause button when making social comments. They are the clumsy, fearless, accident-prone kids who bump into walls, fall off tables and run across roads without looking. In the early school years, they are the fun, precocious children with lots of fans. By Year 2 at school they are the boisterous, annoying children who find it hard to keep friends.

The media focuses on hyperactive ADHD – kids who are physically overactive, disruptive and unpredictable. These are not 'naughty' kids, yet the public perception is that they are the products of 'bad' parents. We need to change this public mindset.

How is ADHD diagnosed?

ADHD is a clinical diagnosis made by a doctor or psychologist. There is no blood test or special way to confirm this condition. A paediatrician takes a history of a child's problems with concentration, learning, socialising and behaviour. Medical, social and emotional causes of distractibility and hyperactivity are excluded before a diagnosis of ADHD is confirmed.

A variety of standardised questionnaires such as the Conners and the SWAN Rating Scale screen to see if a child meets the criteria for having ADHD. *DSM-5* criteria are the most formal way of assessing ADHD.

DSM-5 *criteria*

Most Australian doctors use the American Psychiatric Association *DSM-5* criteria to make this diagnosis. This is a series of eighteen questions: nine of which ask about inattention and nine about hyperactivity and impulsivity. They ask if your child has problems listening, getting organised or following instructions. They question if your child fidgets, talks a lot and interrupts conversations.

Many 'normal' children do these things some of the time. Children with ADHD do them a lot. To have ADHD, a child has to demonstrate a persistent pattern of at least six inattentive or hyperactive and impulsive behaviours in more than one setting. This can be at school and home. These behaviours impair a child's daily functioning and development. They have a significant academic and social effect. You can search on the internet for the *DSM-5* diagnostic criteria if you want more information.

The Conners questionnaire

The Conners 3rd Edition consists of a number of rating scales, available in long and short versions, for completion by parents and teachers. It is available in hard copy and online formats and for self-rating by adolescents. Comorbid (accompanying) conditions such as anxiety, depression, learning difficulty, social problems and oppositional behaviours can also be identified. The clinical progress of children commenced on stimulant medication for ADHD can be monitored. Schools and clinical psychologists often use this clinical tool.

SWAN Rating Scale

Other screening questionnaires include the SWAN Rating Scale for ADHD, adapted from James M. Swanson, PhD, from the University of California. This has eighteen questions covering inattentive and hyperactive behaviours.

Brain imaging

Fancy and expensive brain scans such as SPECT (Single Photon Emission Computer Tomography) scans are not routinely done in children. They don't add value to the clinical diagnosis of ADHD.

Brain studies done in selected cohorts of children with ADHD have reported changes such as thinning of the outer or cortical parts of the front of the brain. This is one area of the brain that controls attention span, self-regulation and motor activity. The good news is that the brain can change. In these same studies, children whose ADHD improved during adolescence and early adulthood showed an increase in brain tissue on follow-up scans in the right parietal lobe, another area that controls attention.

IQ tests

Psychometric tests assess our intelligence quotient or IQ. They can support the clinical diagnosis of ADHD. The Wechsler Intelligence Scale for Children – Fourth Edition (WISC-IV) is an IQ test that assesses language and visual learning skills. It can be used in children from 6 years of age. The more recent version of this test is now available – the WISC-V.

Children with ADHD have identified strengths and weaknesses on IQ testing. Working memory and processing speed, indicators of executive functioning, tend to score lower in children with ADHD and learning disorders than students without those problems.

Working memory and processing speed

Working memory is the brain's 'to-do list'. Some brains have space to record only a few items. This makes the recall of instructions difficult. They could do with more RAM. Your genes determine processing speed. It's a bonus if you're given a fast computer-processing chip. A slow chip means you need more 'think time', even if you are really smart.

Emotional IQ

Most young children have a developmental lag between their emotional IQ, which is the ability to reason, empathise and self-settle, and their intellectual capacity, or cognitive IQ. Typical screaming matches in 2 and 3 year olds are part of normal development. A young child is still developing their emotional IQ skills. Early tantrums don't mean ADHD. As children develop vocabulary and the ability to use language to problem-solve they don't need to use emotional outbursts as their primary form of communication.

Children with language difficulties due to autism, selective mutism or complex language disorders can have persistent emotional outbursts as they progress through school. So too can very bright but socially immature children. They can be viewed as 'problem' children and falsely assigned a label of ADHD.

Gifted kids

Intellectually gifted students can have excellent working memory and processing speed skills, but present with ADHD characteristics because their brain is literally 'buzzing'. Their inquisitive minds seek knowledge. They ask numerous questions, interrupt and are often active and 'on the go'. When very young, their emotional and social IQ drags behind their strong cognitive IQ. This mismatch makes them appear impulsive, emotionally intense, volatile and inattentive. These kids do best with a laterally thinking and creative teacher who 'gets' them. Treating them for ADHD can make them worse.

Medical screening

Testing vision and hearing is important to make sure that a child can see and hear! A blood test can exclude a thyroid gland problem. Low blood sugar levels can affect concentration. Low iron affects concentration and learning. A sleep study may demonstrate restlessness, described as a periodic limb movement disorder or sleep apnoea.

An electroencephalogram (EEG) excludes small recurrent seizures seen in absence seizures, a form of epilepsy. These used to be called petit mal fits. They can be hard to distinguish from daydreaming spells. They affect concentration and school progress.

It is important that paediatricians ask about family dynamics, including recent separation and possible protective issues. A diagnosis of ADHD in a child who is the victim of domestic violence needs to be made with great caution. These children are stressed and present with erratic and difficult behaviours, peer issues and school failure.

Risk factors for ADHD?

Having a parent, grandparent or sibling with diagnosed ADHD is a common 'risk factor'. A diagnosis is more likely in boys.

Genetic syndromes such as Turner, Klinefelter, Prader-Willi, Smith–Magenis, velocardiofacial (22q.11.2 deletion), Angelman, Williams and Fragile X are associated with ADHD. You won't be familiar with these conditions, but will know about autism.

Children with autism and the genetic condition Fragile X syndrome (FXS) are more likely to have ADHD. I have discussed FXS under the section on autism. It is a genetic disorder, more common in boys than girls, associated with intellectual and learning problems and specific physical characteristics.

Foetal alcohol spectrum disorder

When a pregnant mother smokes, her unborn child is exposed to a toxic environment and is at risk of developing ADHD in childhood. There are similar concerns about prenatal exposure to alcohol. Foetal alcohol spectrum disorder (FASD) is linked to children whose mothers consumed alcohol at a vulnerable time of foetal growth during their pregnancy. Many would say, at any time during pregnancy.

These children have the physical, behavioural and cognitive changes induced by alcohol, even in small amounts. They include subtle facial and head shape abnormalities, low IQ and developmental, learning and behavioural problems such as ADHD.

This diagnosis requires a special assessment. There is no simple clinical screening test that local doctors or community and private paediatricians can do.

Preterm birth

Prematurity, low birth weight and head trauma are implicated but unproven risk factors of ADHD. A Western Australian study, by Silva, D. et al. (2015), has found that prematurity increases the already greater association of learning problems in children with ADHD. Around 25 per cent of boys and girls with ADHD are reported as not meeting minimum reading standards by Year 7. Girls with ADHD are said to be more impaired in numeracy than their male peers with ADHD.

ADHD comorbidity

A number of conditions occur with ADHD and make it worse. They include anxiety (20 to 30 per cent), depression (33 per cent) and learning disorders (20 to 60 per cent). Language-based learning disorders are linked more to the inattentive and combined presentation of ADHD than hyperactive ADHD. Dysgraphia, a specific learning disorder of written expression, often complicates ADHD, particularly in boys.

Kids with ADHD frequently have hypermobility of their joints. This makes it hard for them to write for long periods. They have motor-planning problems, which really just means 'clumsy'. The proper name is developmental coordination disorder (DCD) or developmental dyspraxia. The term DAMP (Deficits in Attention, Motor control and Perception) originated in Sweden and was used to describe 'clumsy' children with attention difficulties.

Significant behavioural disorders, known as oppositional defiant disorder (ODD) and conduct disorder (CD), occur in around a third of cases, most often in ADHD of hyperactive-impulsive and combined types.

How do you treat ADHD?

Consider medication after trying adjunctive therapies. Ensure non-medication interventions are safe and affordable. First sort out parenting issues and address mental health issues including adult anxiety and ADHD.

I observed the behaviour and mood of one child to dramatically improve. I asked his mother whether anything had changed to cause such an emotional shift. She replied, 'Yes, I am now on treatment for ADHD and the house is much calmer and more organised'.

215

Omega-3 fatty acids

Before seeking a medical approach to ADHD, most families trial fish oils and other supplements, gluten-free diets, and sugar- and additive-restricted diets. Fish oil is a source of omega-3 fatty acids. Flaxseed oil contains omega-3 and omega-6 fatty acids. The New Zealand green-lipped mussel is also rich in omega-3 fatty acids. All these extracts are used by parents to manage early ADHD symptoms. Some forms of flaxseed can be toxic, such as immature flaxseed pods or rancid flaxseed oil which has been kept too long or has been affected by light exposure.

Brain training and other approaches

Neurofeedback techniques are being explored to help re-train the brain. This is a behaviour therapy program reported to have some benefits for inattention and impulsivity and lesser effects on hyperactivity.

Parents spend money checking vision and hearing, trying visual tracking exercises, computer brain programs, kinesiology and electrical brain activity studies or hair analysis studies. They are often desperate and fatigued when they speak to a doctor about trialling stimulant medication for their child's ADHD.

There are many ways to manage ADHD. I have included some practical resources that detail options for parents in the reference section on ADHD. Strategies include education and behavioural support, clinical psychology intervention, life skill coaches and modifying lifestyle. The practice of mindfulness has become more popular as a holistic approach to ameliorate the emotional outbursts of some children with ADHD.

Stimulants are just one option. They always work much better in combination with other therapies and supports.

Stimulant medication used in ADHD

Medical treatment of ADHD with stimulant medication is an option when ADHD affects a child's academic, behavioural, emotional or social functioning. Sometimes medication helps a lot, particularly in children with hyperactive and impulsive ADHD.

Stimulant medications used in the management of ADHD include methylphenidate (Ritalin, Ritalin LA and Concerta) and dexamphetamine (short-acting, compounded) and sustained-release lisdexamfetamine dimesilate, (Vyvanse). An alternative medication is the non-stimulant atomoxetine (Strattera).

We don't understand exactly how these medications work. But, we know that they can affect the balance of chemicals called neurotransmitters in the brain. These biological substances are involved in executive functions. We need these complex brain actions to think, attend, focus, concentrate, plan, self-motivate and problem-solve.

Methylphenidate and dexamphetamine increase the level of the neurotransmitter dopamine. The non-stimulant atomoxetine increases the levels of dopamine and noradrenaline (norepinephrine).

Stimulant medications have had a role in the medical management of ADHD for more than sixty years. They have a recognised side effect profile with a high margin of safety. Despite their 'bad' image, when prescribed appropriately they can make a positive difference and change the life trajectory of a child.

I will talk more about the use of these medications, their potential benefits and side effects in the childhood section from 5 to 10 years. If your child has early ADHD it is likely to become problematic at this time.

Tics and Tourette Syndrome

Tics are repetitive involuntary muscle movements, which can be associated with ADHD. Motor tics consist of repetitive eye blinking, head nodding, shoulder shrugging or more violent arm and leg movements. They can lessen with age. Tics usually disappear. They persist for some kids and can be problematic.

Vocal tics consist of sounds such as a repetitive cough or throat clearing, or uncommonly the utterance of expletives, called coprolalia.

When multiple motor and vocal tics occur for more than 12 months and commence prior to 18 years of age, they cease being simple tics and are diagnosed as Tourette Syndrome.

Tourette Syndrome can be associated with ADHD, obsessive-compulsive disorder, anxiety, learning disorders, ASD and self-harm. It has an incidence of about 1 per cent and affects boys three to four times more commonly than girls.

Children can suppress their tics for brief periods but will then display a volley of them. Anxiety exacerbates tics. Distraction, such as listening to music or being asleep, settles them. Violent tics or those causing muscle pain need medication.

I saw one boy with severe tics who was able to get rid of them temporarily when he focused on doing maths problems. Other kids find that chewing gum helps. Some clinical psychologists try 'habit reversal' techniques in older kids.

A comprehensive behavioural intervention approach, together with monitored use of medication, is required if the tics are causing discomfort, are frequent or affecting function. A medical opinion from a paediatrician or neurologist is advised.

Central Auditory Processing Disorder (CAPD)

Children with problems hearing, listening, concentrating and learning see an audiologist (hearing specialist). They are diagnosed with a central auditory processing problem (CAPD) or sensory processing problem.

Our brain hears sounds called auditory signals and processes them into meaningful messages. The child who finds it difficult to discriminate sounds may have CAPD. In a noisy classroom they are inattentive, like the child with inattentive ADHD. These two conditions have a very similar clinical presentation. They can be hard to unravel.

How do paediatricians sort out this clinical puzzle? They listen to the child and their family and manage the child's problems. Many of the practical approaches used by teachers to assist the child with ADHD also help the child with CAPD.

From a practical viewpoint, these two conditions are the identical twins of inattention in the classroom. Both can improve with time, life experience and by 'exercising' the brain. I always tell kids that they have to think of their brain like a muscle. If they don't use it, the brain can get lazy and complacent. It loses some of its function and potential.

ADHD – 0 to 5 years

ADHD starts early because of its genetic predisposition. Hyperactive ADHD will be more symptomatic than inattention in the very young child. The child who runs in front of cars and crashes into objects is harder to parent than the daydreaming, quiet one.

We don't treat children under the age of 2 with stimulant medication. It would be uncommon to diagnose ADHD and prescribe medication for behavioural management to a child less than 5 years of age. Early childhood is when you learn to interpret and manage your child's emotional and physical outbursts.

Positive and responsible parenting should be implemented before medication. Fish oil supplements, healthy diets and a good sleep routine can help. Monitoring electronic screen time, especially in very young children, prevents the emotional agitation that can be seen from excessive and prolonged screen use. A household structure and use of visual schedules helps some dysregulated children gain a sense of control and purpose. This helps improve their behaviour.

Children who get bored can suffer with inattention and lack direction. This can lead them to getting into mischief. Engage your child in early play and keep them physically busy so that they are hungry and tired. Read alongside them at bedtime, listen and talk with them. Organise and participate in family activities.

Gluten-free diets

Some parents find that a gluten-free diet helps. People with coeliac disease have a gluten intolerance, which means their gut can't cope with wheat, oats, rye and barley. Corn, rice and almond meal flours are better tolerated.

The FAILSAFE diet

Since the 1970s, Sydney's Prince Alfred Hospital has talked about the FAILSAFE diet and its potential role in behaviour, including ADHD and allergies. This diet is *Free of Additives, Low in Salicylates, Amines and Flavour Enhancers*. Some families adopt this diet or other elimination diets as prescribed by a nutritionist. The FAILSAFE diet cuts out a lot of processed and high-fat foods. It is probably similar to the 'meat and three veg' diet advocated by previous generations!

Medication

A child under 5 years with problematic ADHD may require medication. This should be prescribed by an experienced child psychiatrist or paediatrician to augment behavioural, psychological and parenting input. Criticism of a parent's decision to administer stimulant medication from family, other parents, teachers or professionals is often misinformed and unfounded. It is judgemental and unkind.

ADHD – 5 to 10 years

How it presents

Primary school children with ADHD present early if they have the hyperactive or combined inattentive and hyperactive form of ADHD. They are easily detected within the classroom as the children who fidget, chew their sleeves and collars, bite their nails, doodle on their paper, get up unannounced from their chair or mat and call out.

Socially these kids appear boisterous, precocious and destructive. They invade the personal space of others, physically rush at things, have a poor sense of body position and are accident-prone. These kids can be fun and enthusiastic, particularly in pre-primary and Year 1, but are soon categorised as precocious. By Year 3 they stop getting party invitations and are shunned by other parents in the playground.

School diaries are filled with comments about the negative behaviours of these children. Hyperactive kids are the gas in the bottle, desperate to get out. They will chew their jumper or neck of their tee-shirt. They jiggle their legs. This is often in unison with a parent who will later tell you, 'Maybe I have ADHD too'.

A child with hyperactive ADHD will get out of their seat and climb on a couch or desk when they first meet me. They grab books, toys, pencils, the phone, the blood pressure cuff, scales or anything else that is not tethered down in my room. Some parents, so exhausted by this constant frenetic behaviour, will sit back and wait for me to perform a miracle and to quieten their child. I can't! There is no quick fix. Stimulant medication is not a medical panacea for hyperactivity or inattention. A multimodal approach effects the best outcome.

Inattentive ADHD

The busy or inattentive child is often anxious and overwhelmed. Quiet and overlooked. They fall behind in core learning areas, especially if they also have a language-based learning problem. Comments on their early school reports include words like, 'lacks focus', 'gets distracted', 'needs to be more organised', 'doesn't complete work' and 'requires prompts to finish work'.

Medicating the inattentive child is not a priority, unless despite all other supports they are falling behind academically and struggling socially. Kids with symptomatic ADHD are best treated during the crucial learning years so that they don't fall too far behind prior to high school entry.

A 9-year-old boy with a diagnosis of inattentive ADHD told me that before he was treated for ADHD he couldn't hear his thoughts, especially when the classroom was noisy. He wasn't able to do his work. When he took stimulant medication, he could hear his thoughts.

I respect the decision of parents not to medicate. One mother whose child had ADHD and significant learning disorders told me, 'I can't fix my child, so I am just going to love and enjoy him, the way he is'. She still supported her child's learning needs and encouraged him, but she no longer stressed about her child's learning problems.

I never prescribe medication if the child and parents don't want to trial it, even if I think it would help. This is their decision and sometimes, in severe and problematic ADHD, their consequence.

Benefits of ADHD medication

Children with extreme and early hyperactivity can benefit from stimulant medication such as methylphenidate (Ritalin) and dexamphetamine. It allows them to sit still, focus, listen and complete written work, sometimes for the first time. This makes kids feel more confident and positive about school. They have more success with peer interactions because their 'social filter' works better. Stimulants do not make kids smarter, but when their self-esteem is raised, an improved work ethic results. Teachers and parents become more positive. Then, the student starts to succeed.

The effects of stimulants are immediate, short-lived and positive.

A parent reluctantly started her child on stimulant medication after trying 'everything else'. Her child had been suffering academically and socially. When I reviewed him, the mother cried as she told me what it was like for her child to receive his first birthday invitation.

A medical professional described the positive transformation that stimulant medication had made in her own family. Within twenty minutes of her 10-year-old daughter taking a long-acting stimulant medication, she watched her evolve from a primitive stance of stomping and raging to be the thoughtful and considered child she knew she had.

Another parent expressed regret for having held their child back for so long from a trial of stimulants after seeing the improvement in their child's writing, reading and spelling. They showed me a handwriting sample of messy, disorganised and poorly spaced words scrawled on a few lines before the commencement of stimulant medication. They then displayed a page of neat and creative writing from their child, written whilst on medication.

The best affirmation that stimulant medications help in ADHD is from the child who takes them.

One child told me that on their 'focus tablets' the traffic jam in his head had gone.

A young student told me that being on long-acting stimulant medication was like having a fishing net placed over her head. It trapped all her floating thoughts and ideas and then dragged them back into her head so that she could make sense of them.

I always tell families that the management of ADHD requires a holistic approach. Stimulant medication is just one part. If no one can see a difference from a child taking medication, or if side effects are adverse, then the child stops taking the medication!

Side effects of ADHD medication

Appetite suppression with some initial but transient weight loss is common. Some long-acting stimulants cause more sustained weight loss. Children may eat less lunch, but are usually very hungry at the end of the day. Significant weight loss is not generally problematic. When it is, medication is changed or ceased.

Sleep disturbance occurs more commonly in children with ADHD. Medication can exacerbate this, particularly with long-acting and slow-release stimulant preparations.

Stimulants can increase or decrease anxiety. Some children pick their skin or bite their nails on medication. They start to tic, often presenting as repetitive eye blinking or throat clearing.

Emotional lability can increase on stimulants. Children can be teary or sad as medication wears off – very quiet or withdrawn.

Children diagnosed with autism are exquisitely sensitive to the effects of stimulants. Low doses with small increments are best in this cohort.

Heart problems are a concern to parents. In 2011, *The New England Journal of Medicine* reported no increase in significant cardiac events from stimulant medication taken for the medical management of ADHD in a large cohort of children and young adults from 2 to 24 years of age.

Medication must be ceased if children experience rare side effects of severe depression, agitation or psychosis as manifest by visual or auditory hallucinations.

Rarely, transient visual disturbance and priapism, a painful, persistent penile erection, have been reported.

Up to 80 per cent of children will tolerate stimulant medication with a positive outcome.

Screening tests

An electrocardiogram (ECG) is a printed tracing of the electrical activity of the heart as it contracts. If your child is diagnosed with ADHD, some doctors will order this as a baseline test to confirm a normal heart rhythm.

In Australia, screening tests such as an ECG and blood tests for kidney and liver function are not routinely done prior to commencing stimulants in a healthy child. If your child has a heart murmur, family history of significant or early heart disease, a cardiology opinion is sought from a paediatric heart specialist.

Brain imaging with fancy scans such as MRI (magnetic resonance imaging) and SPECT, a nuclear medicine scan which uses radioactive contrast material, are not routinely done.

Non-stimulant medication and adjunctive treatments

Atomoxetine (Strattera) is a non-stimulant medication prescribed for ADHD. It is helpful for inattentive ADHD with anxiety and motor tics and when stimulants cause side effects.

Strattera has to be taken every day and can take eight to twelve weeks before its full effect is realised. Rare side effects of this medication include liver effects and severe depression with suicidal thoughts.

Clonidine is a medication prescribed in very young children with extreme hyperactivity and aggression. They have suspected ADHD but are too young to be given stimulants. In excessive dosage it can cause a dangerous abnormal heartbeat. A baseline ECG may be considered when prescribing this.

There is evidence to support the use of omega-3 fatty acids in ADHD, particularly the hyperactive and impulsive forms. These are found in fish oil. A minimum trial of three months of taking these supplements is recommended. Fish oil may have a small protective benefit in teenagers vulnerable to developing significant mood disorders such as schizophrenia. This is characterised by psychosis – a distortion of reality. Visual and auditory hallucinations and irrational and bizarre behaviours occur.

Parents should be honest with their children about the use of medication. Young children often associate ADHD with 'crazy kids' and perceive this diagnosis as a stigma. Even young children can be upset when told they have ADHD. It is helpful to explain to them what it means to have problems with their concentration and why they are seeing a paediatrician. Some children and teenagers refuse to take medication and we should respect their decision.

Antidepressant and atypical antipsychotic medication

Antidepressants and very occasionally antipsychotic medications such as aripiprazole (Abilify) and risperidone (Risperdal) are prescribed for children with severe anxiety and depression. These potent medications are also used in the treatment of adult schizophrenia.

Antidepressants known as selective serotonin reuptake inhibitors (SSRIs) are prescribed by child and adolescent psychiatrists and some paediatricians. They assist in the medical management of severe anxiety which impairs the ability of a child to function. They can safely be used in combination with stimulants. There is a slight risk of seizures when used in higher doses with atomoxetine.

Concern has been expressed about increased suicide risk in children and adolescents who take SSRIs. These are prescribed outside the usual age-prescribing outlines and so are considered 'off label' medications. Children and adolescents who are inadequately treated for their anxiety and depression are also at greater risk of suicide.

SSRIs work best when used in combination with cognitive behaviour therapy. A clinical psychologist will assist the child who is anxious or depressed to use their thinking, reasoning and reflective brain to change and control thoughts and actions. They can help a child or adolescent change their learned behavioural response to stressful situations.

Consent

When medication is prescribed, verbal consent from both parents or respective guardians and carers is important. When there is parental separation, written consent from both parents is advisable before prescribing stimulants. If there are imminent court and custodial procedures, it is not appropriate to commence stimulant medication.

In Australia the prescription of stimulants is well regulated by some state health authorities. This is for the safety and benefit of doctors and patients. Some countries are seen to overprescribe stimulant medication.

ADHD and oppositional behaviours

If a child under 10 years has impulsive behaviours that brand them as early troublemakers they are at risk of developing more serious oppositional, defiant and conduct disorders ODD and CD. These diagnoses describe children who steal, are pathological liars, light fires and bully. They are socially displaced. We love these kids, but they are hard to like. We need to engage professional help to change their life trajectory.

We need these kids to engage with our education system, to be literate and learn. If we fail to manage disruptive, emotionally dysregulated and socially deviant behaviours early, we can't expect our police commissioners to fix them later. We don't want these kids to fall into the realm of the juvenile justice system, but some will. Their failure is our failure.

ADHD and teachers

In primary school, parents should liaise with their child's teacher when a diagnosis of ADHD has been made. Some parents choose not to do this if they perceive the teacher to have a judgemental attitude about ADHD.

Many teachers suspect that a student has ADHD or suggest this diagnosis, particularly when hyperactivity is present. Kids with ignored ADHD suffer academically and socially. They get sad, anxious, mad and bad. They lose their sense of belonging.

Children with ADHD can have learning difficulties, social problems, anxiety, depression, and autism. They require a whole team approach. This consists of family, teachers, education assistants, occupational therapists, speech pathologists, physiotherapists, clinical psychologists, social workers, counsellors and life skill coaches. They benefit from ongoing management from their medical practitioner, paediatricians, and child and adolescent psychiatrists.

ADHD learning styles

Children with ADHD tend to be strong visual and hands-on learners rather than auditory or listening ones.

A mother saw the visual learning strength in her child with ADHD. He had poor muscle tone, joint laxity and problems with muscle coordination, called dyspraxia. He was struggling to coordinate his swimming strokes required for butterfly kick. She conferred with his swimming teachers and suggested that they video his strokes to demonstrate what he was doing. She asked them to show him a video of the correct technique for butterfly kick. Once her child had seen the videos he jumped back in the water and swam with the correct kick!

Kids with ADHD can be very creative, musical or artistic. Many are great at drums and percussion instruments. This group of kids can see and conceptualise whole concepts. They give a correct or nearly correct answer to maths problems but struggle to demonstrate the steps taken to achieve their task.

'Chalk and talk' teaching is when the teacher writes and speaks when giving students new information. It is difficult for the child with ADHD to learn with this teaching method. These students do better when they receive visual prompts and can 'divide and conquer' their workload by tackling small amounts of work at a time.

Written assessment and the pressure of time limits create high levels of anxiety for students with ADHD. They struggle to succeed in what they perceive as a hostile learning environment. They are best assessed on oral presentation and when given extra think time for verbal responses in the classroom.

Homework during the early school years is a battle and won't be done. Insisting that it will destroys the love of learning and a parent's sanity.

Students with ADHD need a compassion-focused approach by parents and teachers. They thrive when they meet a teacher who 'gets' them and doesn't judge.

ADHD and learning disorders

Inattentive ADHD is frequently complicated by language and social problems and the specific learning disorders, dyslexia (reading), dyscalculia (math) and dysgraphia (writing and spelling). Joint hypermobility, low muscle tone, fatigue and clumsiness are common and impact on writing speed and neatness. These conditions limit the amount of written work produced.

The School Curriculum and Standards Authority in each state and territory will allow special considerations such as extra time or 'concentration' breaks for students with learning problems.

Working memory

Children with ADHD, particularly with comorbid inattention or learning disorders, have problems with working memory. This function stores the brain's 'to-do list' and works through and acts upon it.

Some kids become asymptomatic or can manage their inattentive ADHD as they mature. Young adults diagnosed with ADHD in childhood learn to utilise electronic planners, lists, and gain organisational and life skills. This can help them function competently without medication. Some still benefit from the prescribed use of stimulants as adults.

There is an emerging market for tools and electronic programs devised to improve working memory such as Cogmed and Jungle Memory. I have listed website details in the resources section.

I won't comment medically on the efficacy or long-term benefit of these programs. If a child is keen to trial something that is safe, affordable and doesn't impact negatively on their play or learning time, give it a go. Many families provide positive feedback on these programs which target the building of visual memory.

The neuroplasticity of the brain means that working memory can improve. You can't as easily change the genetic hardware that gives some kids a slow processing speed. These kids struggle to take in visual and auditory information quickly. They need extra think time, written and visual prompts and benefit from learning by rote (repetition).

Improving working memory

There are some simple, cost-free and practical ways of developing working memory. When I was a child, rote learning was utilised, particularly in relation to times tables. Singing sequencing songss such as 'ten green bottles hanging on the wall' and 'I spy', used to be classic car travel games for young children. Whilst very trying for parents, they were great early memory games for children. Some kids learn best by the recall of rhyme, which is why Dr Seuss books have found a new niche. They teach kids to read using rhyme, repetition, phonics and fun.

> *When I was walking along a street shopping strip, I passed a man and his young daughter walking towards the fruit shop. This dad was giving his 5-year-old daughter a free working memory exercise. He said, 'Now remember we have to buy polony, oranges, watermelon, eggs, rice and salami'. Then he said, 'Now remind me what we are buying', and she replied correctly.*

You might want to think about how you would remember that list. The acronym 'POWERS' would work.

Other people might choose auditory recall to repeat the list. Setting the words to song can help, as can visualising the food in your mind. Mnemonics are also useful memory aids. My favourite was 'my very eager mate just swept up nine pins'. This gave me the correct sequence of Mercury, Venus, Earth, Mars, Jupiter, Saturn, Uranus, Neptune and Pluto from the sun.

Teachers understand the importance of visual cues and learning tips. They encourage students to colour-code thcir subject folders or use colour highlighters to plan study time for each subject on a visual schedule or diary.

If kids remember 'best' in pictures, they could try thinking about a super sandwich made up of all the items on a shopping list. I suggest they start with four things and try to build up to ten. A shopping list with carrots, onions, grapes, bread and spaghetti can be recalled by picturing a carrot hula hooping with an onion ring. Imagine the carrot looking at the scene with big grape eyes whilst balanced on top of a loaf of bread which is precariously balanced on a strand of spaghetti. I bet you didn't think shopping with a child could be so much fun!

Neil MacKay's book *Taking the Hell Out of Homework* outlines a number of practical learning strategies for students with dyslexia and weakness in working memory.

If my child has ADHD, will they have it as an adult?
As many as 60 per cent of children affected by ADHD will have some features of ADHD in adulthood. Not all adult ADHD, particularly if uncomplicated, will require ongoing treatment. The positive news is that the brain has some flexibility or neuroplasticity. As long as the brain is used, it can improve.

When a child has persistent traits of inattention, hyperactivity and impulsivity, it is safer for them to remain on stimulant medication as an adolescent and emerging adult. This applies to driving and working in high-risk areas with electricity or on building and mining sites.

All about specific learning disorder (SLD)

'Normal' children find it hard to read, spell, write and do maths. I tell kids who struggle to learn that I can't play the clarinet very well. Everyone finds something 'tricky'. Young children wish schoolwork was easier. The favourite part of the school day for these children is recess and lunchtime. For kids with learning problems, no time of the day is fun.

The *DSM-5* classifies specific learning disorder as a problem with reading, writing or maths. Previously SLD was referred to as a specific learning disability. Specific learning disorder is an impairment with written expression (dysgraphia), reading (dyslexia) or mathematics (dyscalculia).

Dyslexia

Most families have heard about dyslexia, an impairment in reading, that is unexpected for measured intellectual capacity. By definition, a child with a high IQ but below average reading age has dyslexia.

Dyslexia can be associated with inattentive ADHD. This diagnosis can be made when a child has reached the age of around 8 years. It can stigmatise a child. Although an unhelpful label, it facilitates access to additional school help.

Dyslexia occurs in around 5 to 12 per cent of school-age children. It is caused by an impairment in phonological processing. This means the child's ability to understand letter-sound relationships. Students with dyslexia have problems decoding words, reading fluently and later with reading comprehension.

You can have dyslexia and still succeed academically. A number of talented actors have disclosed their battle with dyslexia.

Kids with dyslexia have a problem with reading but not with their smartness. Acknowledge that reading will be hard work for them. Avoid forcing them to read.

Alternative reading methods

Reading can become a chore for these students. Keep it fun. Suggest audio or talking books, alongside reading and conversation. Some families explore alternative learning interventions such as the Irlen Method. This uses coloured lenses to assist a child's eye tracking and reading. I don't get involved in these family-based decisions. If a child is prepared to undertake a learning program, which is safe and a reasonable cost, we should support them. If something works for your child, do it!

I endorse a no homework or a limited homework policy for students with dyslexia in the first three years of primary school. Learning-affected children and their families already do extra work with tutors, speech pathologists and occupational therapists. When they escape school they need time to play.

Families make drastic lifestyle changes to support their child's dyslexia or other learning disorders. They relocate the whole family interstate or overseas to access an intense teaching program such as the Arrowsmith Program. This has been implemented in a number of schools in Canada, the US, New Zealand, Australia and Malaysia.

Before making significant lifestyle changes, seek professional advice from a clinical psychologist or child psychiatrist. Whilst big decisions are the prerogative of parents, advocacy for the child warrants objective input to assist in the transition or timing of them.

Children with high functioning autism and learning problems transition poorly when moving home or school. Siblings can find enforced change detrimental to their social and emotional development. Parental relationship may be compromised.

Standardised testing

It is not fair that children with severe dyslexia have to pass onerous and regular standardised tests in literacy. This just confirms how challenging reading is for these children. It doesn't incite them to learn.

Special consideration

Having a learning problem does not automatically get you extra help or support at school. This is a great frustration for parents, teachers and students. A diagnosis of an intellectual disability, autism spectrum disorder or mental health disorder by a child psychiatrist will gain eligibility for some extra education assistance.

If a student has dysgraphia, they require a written report from an occupational therapist or clinical psychologist to be eligible for extra time, use of a computer or support with a scribe.

Developmental coordination disorder or developmental dyspraxia can qualify a student for extra time. This label has to come from a clinical psychologist or occupational therapist. These children find it hard to tie shoelaces, colour in and cut with scissors. They have poor ball-throwing skills.

You will need to check with your school and the state or territory's School Curriculum and Standards Authority equivalent for eligibility criteria and required documentation.

Dysgraphia

Dysgraphia is characterised by spelling, grammar and handwriting problems. Handwriting difficulty is also categorised as a developmental coordination disorder. This describes children who have problems with fine motor skills such as penmanship and the 'clumsy child' with gross motor problems.

Dysgraphia is quite common in kids with inattentive ADHD and has a significant impact on their marks in English and subjects which require written responses. It occurs in about 7 to 15 per cent of school-age children. These kids can be competent with oral presentation and verbal answers. Some schools recognise this and accommodate these creative and intellectually sound students. They allow them to use laptops for classroom work.

Dysgraphia can be due to problems with motor planning which makes it difficult for a student to express their thoughts in written form. It can refer to the mechanics of writing or both. Most kids can tell you what is 'tricky' about their writing.

Students with dysgraphia have difficulties with spelling and grammar, poor spatial orientation of letters and mix printing and cursive writing. They have unfinished and omitted words. Handwriting is slow, messy or illegible, disorganised and limited.

I suggest to these kids that they do lots of 'talking work' at home, download a typing program, become touch typists and invest in speech recognition software programs.

Most problems come in multiples. If you have dysgraphia, you are more likely to be a boy with inattentive ADHD, subtle language-based learning problems and hypermobile (loose and floppy) joints. This makes handwriting a chore. Fatigability of pencil grip is common and work avoidance understandable.

Dyscalculia

Dyscalculia (maths disorder) is a chronic, lifelong learning disorder (LD). Understanding and learning arithmetic can be particularly taxing. The language of maths, such as reading and comprehending worded problems, can also be hard. Dyscalculia occurs in around 6 per cent of children.

Nonverbal learning disorder

Nonverbal learning disorder describes a cluster of symptoms often seen in children diagnosed with HFA with Asperger presentation. These students have good basic language skills but as they progress through school they have problems with higher-order reading, inferential language and social reasoning. They have good rote skills, and cope with early reading and spelling, but find maths hard and struggle with visual-spatial tasks. They have problems with attention and concentration and are diagnosed with ADHD. Anxiety and depression are common comorbidities.

Language-based learning disorder

Language-based learning disorder presents with problems in reading and writing. It coexists with dyslexia and dysgraphia. These students have stronger visual than aural skills. They struggle with vocabulary, phonological awareness (discriminating the sounds in words), grammar, narrative and conversational speech.

Learning disorders are present at birth or acquired after birth in the case of brain infections, such as encephalitis (brain inflammation), or severe meningitis and brain injury. Some medical and genetic conditions, including chromosomal disorders like Fragile X syndrome have intellectual and learning disabilities. Developmental conditions including ADHD, autism, anxiety and depression can also affect cognition and learning.

There can be a family history of learning disorders, especially dyslexia and ADHD, and mental health morbidity due to anxiety, depression and bipolar disorder. Language-based learning problems can be associated with some cases of inattentive ADHD.

The importance of a stimulating, nurturing and literacy-rich early learning environment cannot be underestimated. Studies in the UK have shown that children under the age of 3 years from a language-poor home are behind in their vocabulary compared with students who enter the school system from a language-rich environment. Many don't catch up.

Language needs to be practised. Parents should read with their young children, talk, play and listen to them. Electronic screens cannot effect this role. Learning from a touch screen is lazy learning. Excessive screen time may impede early language development. It prevents kids using language to problem-solve.

Happy, emotionally resilient children with supportive social scaffolding are primed to learn when they enter the school system. All children, particularly those with a specific learning disorder, require adequate social, emotional, fine motor, gross motor and problem-solving skills to be school ready. This optimises their learning. Parents must help their children attain these tools.

The choice of school for the child with learning disorders needs careful consideration and is best made on the basis of emotional and social 'best fit' and not on academic grounds alone.

SLD – 0 to 5 years

Childhood development is a continuum along which pivotal milestones are achieved, but at different ages and stages, dependent on the child. The child with early global developmental delay (GDD) may receive a later diagnosis of specific learning disorder or intellectual disability.

SLDs can't be diagnosed definitively before 8 years of age. Prior to this age, a child is vulnerable to developing dyslexia, dysgraphia, dyscalculia or nonverbal learning problems.

A child has global developmental delay if their developmental or functional ability is at least twelve months behind their chronological age in two or more of the five domains of child development. These are social and emotional development, language and communication, fine motor and coordination ability, gross motor function and performance, and cognitive and reasoning function.

Children with developmental dyspraxia can have early delay but often show catch up in their development.

All children should be valued and treated as having potential during their early years. This is the time when early intervention has its greatest impact. It is helpful for parents to focus their energies on the needs of their child during these early years, rather than seeking diagnoses and causes. Expensive investigations such as microarray chromosome tests show minor genetic abnormalities in the 'normal' child. Mostly, we can't give parents an answer as to why their child has a learning or intellectual problem.

Genetic screening

Sometimes chromosome testing is warranted, particularly if a child has autism or dysmorphic features. Dysmorphism means that a person's physical appearance is unusual. Clusters of 'different' facial, hand and feet features can be seen in genetic disorders such as Fragile X syndrome. This is associated with learning or intellectual disability, ADHD and autism.

There are some genetic mutations thought to be linked with learning problems. It is not always helpful to identify these in families, particularly if a further diagnosis doesn't alter the child's management. The genetic condition myotonic dystrophy can have an onset in adulthood. It is not advisable to test for it in childhood. This diagnosis could have insurance and other implications.

Parental consent for the genetic testing of some medical conditions, particularly those appearing in later life, removes the opportunity for the older child to be involved in decisions that involve testing of their genetic material.

SLD – 5 to 10 years

Read with your child

Early learning problems can be missed by parents and teachers. Literacy problems present in the school Years 5 to 7.

One of the reasons for missing the gaps in childhood learning is that parents and educators have been too busy to teach the traditional three 'Rs' of writing, reading and arithmetic. Teachers acknowledge that the early school curriculum is too cluttered. Parents are swamped by commitment to extracurricular activities for their children. Rote learning and phonics are shunned. Families are increasingly complex. Kids take their emotional problems to school. Autism rates have gone up. ADHD makes learning harder.

Electronic screens have displaced blackboards, whiteboards and teachers. They have created a classroom environment of 'lazy learning'. Some screen time can be relaxing for children, especially those with autism or ADHD, but too much can promote aggression and decrease problem-solving ability. Young children who live in time-poor or literacy-poor homes can become dependent or even addicted to screen time. This can affect their language development.

Childhood educational TV programs such as *Play School* and *Sesame Street* encourage the use of vocabulary and language, but others don't. Nothing beats talking and reading with your child every day.

Busy homes

Children are sent to school tired, dirty, hungry, sad, angry and anxious. They don't always have their recess or lunch. Teachers feel obliged to spend their own money to purchase food for them. Children are dropped off early and picked up late. They are unsupervised within the school grounds.

Many private schools have the advantage of paid, structured before and after school services, breakfast, sports and homework clubs and early starts. This is helpful for working parents without extended family support. However, you have to be able to afford these services.

Funding flexible working hours for teachers and education assistants within the government system would make sense. Most nursing shifts commence at 7 am. This reflects the pace set by surgeons who historically have always started operating early. This is not conducive to raising children easily. Nor are night shifts.

Busy classrooms

Children with ADHD and those with autism get overwhelmed in the visually busy classroom. Yet, most primary school classrooms are set up like obstacle courses. You have to duck and weave your way through bits of hanging paper, string, ribbons and coloured cardboard. Teachers seem to be rated on how much clutter they can fit into their room rather than their ability to teach.

Reading books can be similarly busy. Students with ADHD find number and word clutter on a page confusing. The challenge for teachers is to cater for the learning needs, preferences and styles of each student.

Teaching methods

My kids went through a school system where early literacy was 'caught', like the common cold. Spelling was taught with a mixture of methods, dependent on the teacher assigned to your child's class. Spelling was approached using a number of systems, including THRASS, Smart Words, basic phonics or thematic spelling lists. I didn't have a clue what was going on.

THRASS is an acronym for 'Teaching Handwriting, Reading, and Spelling Skills'. It incorporates an innovative phonics teaching style. Thematic spelling involves putting lists of words together based on subject matter and not on phonetic similarity. Kids get a list of theme words such as stars, sun, moon and comet to learn. This makes no sense to me unless your child has a capacious working memory. This pretty much wipes out most kids with ADHD.

Smart Words was a program introduced to my kids in the primary school years. My understanding of it was that it used spelling rules, grouped words and word patterns to help children use phonetics and think cognitively to retain long-term spelling strategies.

If your child misses the basic building blocks of spelling and grammar, they will present later with literacy and grammar problems. If they don't spend time spelling, they won't be able to spell! I am not blaming teachers for these gaps which I have seen repeatedly over nearly twenty years. It is a systems fault. We all need to correct this. Parents must continue to support and trust their child's teacher.

The challenge of learning disorders

Children who have dyslexia, dysgraphia or ADHD need extra help, support and understanding to assist them with spelling, reading, writing and grammar. There is no point in making these children take home unfinished worksheets. It is cruel to keep them away from their peers and play at recess or lunch so that they finish work. They can't do it yet! They are not lazy, naughty or poorly motivated. They are children with specific learning disorders. They are often anxious, avoidant under-achievers. It is our job as parents and teachers to be patient, kind, creative, and innovative in our teaching and adopt a nurturing approach towards them.

A 9-year-old boy with high functioning autism, ADHD and anxiety was home schooled by his mother. He had been bullied at his mainstream school and forced to stay in class at recess and lunchtime to complete work. He had been failing school.

He told me that he was happy at home and proudly showed me his writing book. 'Look at my story', he said with a huge smile. 'My mum said, the most I had to write each day was one page. At my old school I was so stressed that I couldn't write anything. Now I love writing'.

Children with ADHD, autism, learning disorders and anxiety suffer with performance anxiety. They respond well to setting limits on work expectations. This gives them the opportunity to succeed and the incentive to keep trying.

Our education system assesses children for what they don't know, rather than getting kids to divulge what they have learned. A child may tell you about a topic, but is unable to express their knowledge in writing. Why don't we test these students on their visual and oral strengths?

Children with severe dyslexia face failure repeatedly through school. In Western Australia they are tested for numeracy and literacy skills in pre-primary. They sit NAPLAN (National Assessment Program – Literacy and Numeracy) standardised tests in Years 3, 5, 7 and 9. They have the unrelenting pressure of failing school graduation if they can't pass their Year 9 NAPLAN test or subsequent OLNA (Online Literacy and Numeracy Assessment) to a satisfactory level.

How many bright, creative, competent students do we penalise? This education policy needs review.

Students with SLDs need to focus on the core learning areas of numeracy and literacy and emotional and social skills during the early school years.

Maths and English competency gives a student choice. Parents and teachers support the student with learning problems by providing a positive learning environment and engaging with them. The gifted teacher is able to reach out and connect to these difficult and complex students.

Education screening

Paediatricians are asked to assess the developmental and intellectual ability of children of 4 and 5 years of age. This can assist parents and teachers make decisions about appropriate early education placements for children who have global developmental delay, significant language problems or autism. School psychologists can conduct formal IQ testing on students once they have reached 6 years of age on a priority basis.

Griffiths assessment

Paediatricians use a number of developmental screening tools to work out at what developmental level a child is functioning.

Some paediatricians have experience using the Griffiths Mental Development Scales – Revised assessment of children from 0 to 2 years and the Griffiths Mental Development Scales – Extended Revision (GMDS-ER) from 2 to 8 years. Or the new Griffiths III.

This is a useful screening tool but should not be equated with an IQ test. It is language-weighted and dependent on examiner competency and parent report. It is not a reliable test for children with developmental dyspraxia who have early language problems and fine and gross motor coordination difficulties.

IQ tests

School psychologists use standardised IQ testing. The Wechsler Preschool and Primary School Intelligence – Third Edition (WPPSI-III) – Australian IQ test assesses children from 2 years and 6 months to 7 years and 3 months.

The Wechsler Intelligence Scale for Children – Fourth Edition (WISC-IV) and revised WISC-V tests the intelligence of children from the age of 6 years until early adulthood.

Some psychologists use the Stanford-Binet Intelligence Scales – Fifth Edition for assessing cognitive intelligence. This tool can be used in children from as young as 2 years and in adults. It is a good test to detect early intellectual giftedness.

Nonverbal IQ tests are used when a child has a significant language problem or when English is a second language. Tests include the Leiter-R (Revised), applicable from the age of 2 years to 20 years and 11 months, and the Wechsler Nonverbal Scale of Ability (WNV). Details of these and other standardised psychometric assessments performed by registered psychologists are beyond the scope of this discourse.

IQ tests are affected by the child's ability to concentrate. They are adversely affected by fatigue, illness or if a child dislikes or is fearful of the examiner. They do not test for values of kindness, patience, tolerance, compassion, understanding, emotional or social resilience. Nor for creativity, motivation or aspiration. There is a consensus that a child's academic results are determined more by their emotional intelligence, the ability to self-reflect, motivate and learn than by raw cognitive intelligence.

The paediatrician's role

Schools need paediatric input for vulnerable students in kindergarten and pre-primary. They seek a medical opinion as to whether a child with academic, social and emotional difficulties has autism, early ADHD or SLD.

Global developmental delay

Most parents know their child's strengths and weaknesses. Paediatricians should listen to their opinions. If a child has a global developmental delay, they are 12 months or more behind in at least two developmental areas. They are at risk of having learning, behavioural and emotional problems upon school entry. If a cognitive lag persists at 5 or 6 years of age, they could have an intellectual disability and will benefit from an education support learning environment. This may be a specialised unit within the school grounds. Children with significant learning problems are stressed by the social and academic challenges of a mainstream class.

Children with significant language difficulty but a normal non-verbal IQ can be referred to a dedicated language centre for the early school years and then attend mainstream schooling.

Medical screening

Students and parents benefit when learning problems are acknowledged. Paediatricians check for any underlying genetic, metabolic, medical, social or emotional reasons for a child's problems.

Eyesight and hearing should be checked. Blood tests are taken to exclude thyroid problems, diabetes, anaemia or liver problems. Urine is tested for rare metabolic diseases and chromosome tests are done to count out an obvious genetic cause for learning problems such as Down syndrome or Fragile X syndrome. Anxiety, depression, bullying, sleep disorders and family disruption can affect early learning. We ask about fits or seizures and for a family history of epilepsy, autism, ADHD or SLD.

Developmental dyspraxia

Children with developmental dyspraxia or DCD can present with delay in their language, fine motor and gross motor abilities. They can present as if they have a significant intellectual delay. Paediatricians need to be very careful in their assessment of these children. They often have hidden cognitive potential. These children can have a form of childhood apraxia of speech. This means they have problems in their speech production with dysfluent speech and impaired planning of language. Intensive and ongoing speech therapy is needed until they are 7 or 8 years of age.

The parental role

Parents source help from multiple agencies when they have a young child with a specific learning disorder. Input is from speech and occupational therapists, physiotherapists, psychologists, life coaches and counsellors, social workers, tutors and teachers. It is important for parents not to overload a child with an intensive learning schedule. Parents need to monitor their child's progress and back off if their child becomes stressed.

The educator's role

There is general concern about the standard of writing, reading, spelling and maths in our children. Parents are frustrated when unable to access sufficient education assistance for children with literacy and numeracy problems.

Children who fall behind in these areas during primary school find it hard to catch up in high school. If they are vulnerable to developing anxiety, they can become work avoidant. ADHD children with learning problems will start to act out and 'play the clown' to deflect their real struggles.

I am respectful of the awesome job and responsibility of educators. Most are dedicated, caring and engage young children to learn. In the early years, educators are part of a system which frustrates them as much as it does parents. We need to encourage gifted and innovative teachers to teach the next generation of Australians.

Some years a child will 'click' with their teacher and have a good year. Other years there is a poor fit between the child and their teacher. Parents will have to work out strategies with their child to get through those years. This prepares a child for the harshness of life outside school.

ADHD and SLD – 10 to 15 years

A bright high school student, now at university, was struggling at an academic selective school and had started to give up. He had cognitive markers and clinical traits of inattentive ADHD. After commencing stimulant medication his grades improved from C's to A's. I recall seeing the change in posture associated with his growing confidence when this student saw me for periodic review. His mother recalled how sad he had been before addressing his ADHD problems.

I reviewed a Year 10 student who was struggling to find the necessary motivation to keep up with her grades, despite her innate brightness. She met the criteria for an inattentive form of ADHD. She had a loving and supportive network and known family history of ADHD. After commencing stimulant medication, she told me that she could focus and do her work. She appeared happy and enthusiastic. Her mother made the statement that treatment had been life-changing for her and commented that her maths grades had gone from 50 per cent to 80 per cent.

ADHD presenting late

Sometimes the older child with ADHD, particularly the very bright student, will present late. Their cognitive strength has enabled them to cruise through the earlier school years, usually with mediocre or even above average marks. They might do well on standardised tests such as NAPLAN in primary school. In secondary school their results can start to decline. Their grades don't always reflect their true academic potential. This is a point of frustration for caring parents and teachers, and for the student.

Students with ADHD can't always accommodate the increased workload and time constraints of assignments and tests as they reach the final high school years. This includes the cohort of kids who are bright, anxious or have autism. If they have a comorbid learning difficulty, especially of written expression, they struggle even more. These students become anxious, depressed and disengaged from school. Sometimes they act out and become one of the labelled troublemakers. This tag may have already followed them from primary school and the earlier high school years.

Diagnosis and treatment

If a clinical diagnosis of ADHD is confirmed in later childhood or adolescence, a trial of stimulant medication can be beneficial – socially and academically.

If a student's ADHD is ignored, they fall further behind academically and socially at school. This could adversely affect their future aspirations.

A medication approach alone is not advocated for the child with ADHD, whatever their developmental stage. There is no value in giving medication if you don't actively address any accompanying learning, emotional or social problems.

Parents can liaise with the school to work out the best education plan for their child. You may have a very bright child with ADHD who is not ready to accept the arduous challenge of academic work required for an ATAR (Australian Tertiary Admission Rank). A vocational training course can provide greater choice for them and enable them to consolidate their learning via alternative pathways. Options include tertiary college, online courses or university entry as a mature-age student or by portfolio entry.

Aim for your child to be happy and graduate, and then support them as they work out their chosen higher education pathway.

I hear parents berate their children for being lazy and throwing away their costly private education. This is not helpful for the child. Education is not about being the best student in the class. It should be about inspiring students to learn so they can convert information into useful knowledge, build friendships, skills and hopes and have purpose when they leave school.

DOs – 5 to 10 years

Do

- teach your child resilience and success through failure
- be a calm, consistent and reflective parent
- provide a safe, secure and nurturing home environment
- ensure healthy eating and sleeping
- maintain the work and lifestyle balance
- avoid a hectic extracurricular schedule
- talk, walk, play and listen to your child
- learn the language of your child from their behaviour
- have electronic screen breaks
- keep up with technology
- avoid electronic, lazy and dismissive parenting
- take charge of childhood anxiety while your child is still young
- be proactive about your own mental health
- keep calm when your child has an emotional meltdown
- act and liaise with the school on physical, social and emotional bullying and cyberbullying
- believe in your child – 110 per cent
- advocate for your child when necessary
- trust, respect and communicate appropriately with your child's teacher

- connect with your local neighbourhood and wider community
- be kind, compassionate, humble and non-judgemental when raising a child
- reconnect with extended family
- ask for help when you need it

DON'Ts – 5 to 10 years

Don't

- adopt time-poor parenting
- demonstrate narcissistic (selfish) parenting
- have controlling and rigid parenting styles
- be inconsistent, erratic and reactive with your parenting
- lack fair, consistent home rules and boundaries
- ignore mental health problems
- forget to listen to your child
- be afraid of your child
- fail to protect your child from emotional, physical and sexual abuse
- emotionally disconnect from your child
- rescue and overprotect your child
- practise 'smother' love

Part 7

Jumping hurdles from 10 to 15

*Unless you're willing to have a go, fail miserably, and
have another go, success won't happen.*

Phillip Adams – Journalist

Transitional years

Changes

Rapid physical growth and emotional change occur from 10 to
15 years of age. The young, compliant child transforms into the
reactive, challenging teenager and newly emerging adult. Your
child is evolving and you have to be prepared to change.

This is a difficult transition time for parents and their adolescent
children. The pre-teen and teen years displace you as a parent.
Pubertal change has great power. Peers become the greatest
influence on your child. Parents learn to step back but not out of
their child's life. This is a time for parenting and not befriending
your child. Don't elevate your child to the role of peer. The less
liked you are by your child, the greater you are loved and respected.

The tween and teen years

Pre-adolescence or the tween time from around 8 to 11 years of age and the teenage years from 12 to 15 are vulnerable years for kids and their parents. A child undergoes physical, physiological, emotional and social growth. It is affected by the fragility of teenage self-esteem, altered body image and a fight for control and independence.

A child leaves the security and structure of primary school to take their place on the high school stage. They enter puberty, change shape and get acne. Girls experience their first period. Hearts are broken and social groups shuffle their boundaries. The mean girls and their meaner mums appear. Online and physical bullying rises and fun and play disappear from the schoolyard.

Friendship groups and interests change, the academic load becomes greater and family dynamics shift. A child embraces their peer group and displaces the family from their confidence.

Social pressures escalate and a gang mentality can replace the simplicity of organised plays and sleepovers. Sexuality is explored and in Years 8, 9 and 10, students are partying with spirits and alcohol on the menu. Years 7, 8 and 9 see the emergence of disordered eating patterns. In Years 9 and 10, self-harm behaviours assume cult status and Years 10, 11 and 12 are known for illicit drug experimentation. There are fortunate families who experience a smooth transition from childhood to adolescence – but not many!

It is vital that parents read the language of their developing adolescent during this time, so that the vulnerable child's anxiety or depression is not overlooked.

Hectic families

The double-digit years from 10 to 15 dictate a new and hectic pace of parenting. Unresolved problems from earlier childhood become problematic. Parents raising children with the added burden of social media commentary face challenges unknown to earlier generations of parents.

The most common complaint from parents is that children are highly anxious, life is complex, too busy and that they are time-poor. Many of us wish the lives of our children away, instead of embracing failure and disappointment with vigour and enjoying a moment from each day.

As parents we have choices. We need to slow down and simplify life. This means making the hard decisions and being the parent. We don't have to accept the disempowerment of parenthood. Until parents stop playing the victim, we won't shift our social trajectory.

Parents can make micro changes in the way they parent. They can introduce an electronic curfew for young children after five o'clock at night, or insist on regular family meal times. These actions facilitate positive family social connections. Time to communicate with your child is the cheapest and most effective form of therapy. We struggle to effect this.

Some parents choose denial, distraction and drink to blot out their parental responsibility. Unresolved issues from a troubled childhood impact on a parent's ability to provide a secure emotional and financial base for their own child. Community, friends, family, neighbours and professional bodies and resources have to step up and help.

Reality parenting

It is difficult to live a private life in a busy suburban street. Social media pervades homes. Kids today are much more relaxed about privacy rights than their parents. They are yet to learn the implications of impulsive and reckless digital postings. These can affect them later as professional adults working in areas of education, law, medicine and the public service.

The child and pre-adolescent years are watched and scrutinised by neighbours, schools, friends and families with as much vigour as a reality TV show. Just put on the blinkers. Don't get distracted from your parental duty of care. Provide the best home environment that you can for your child.

There will be occasions when you find yourself in crisis and need to be bailed out by professional help. Never be embarrassed. Many other imperfect families surround you.

Time-poor parenting

Most parents describe the preteen and teenage years as difficult. At times they tiptoe around the difficult teenage issues to avoid conflict. We have all done this. My way of coping with these tiptoe years was to take life slowly, in two-second instalments. My kids can attest to my habitual response to their question of 'When can you take me?' being 'In two seconds'. There was never enough time. I recall some wise words from Jo Court, the wife of an ex-premier of Western Australia. Her words were to the effect that 'For children to have quality time, they need quantity of time'.

In our family, time was always in deficit. Excuses were common. We found it difficult to say 'No' to our children. Like many families, we struggled to balance time spent on work, play and organised extracurricular activities. The onerous commitment to these activities sometimes influenced the structure and function of family life.

This is a trap for many loving and well-meaning families. Our society of excess allows too many choices. Parents want to give their children the sporting, drama and music opportunities that they didn't have.

Life balance

When choosing an extracurricular activity for your child first ask yourself what your child wants to do. It is about them – not you! A child needs to find their own place and sense of belonging with your parental guidance and support.

Where sibling rivalry is problematic, address it and consider different pathways for your children. This means they don't compete against one another, which is particularly relevant for twin siblings or siblings close in age. When this is not possible, be fair and just in the way you distribute your parental time commitment and the interest you take in their hobbies.

During the primary school years and in early high school, encourage your child to have a go at something. Children need to learn through failure to achieve success. It helps the physical, emotional and social health of a child to participate in a summer and a winter sport.

Prior to high school entry, kids cope with two or even three different activities. These include sport, music, tutoring, drama, art or Scouts. In secondary school, drop back to two extra interests, and by Year 10 and 11 to just one. That is unless sport, music and drama are part of your child's school curriculum load.

If your child is a gifted student and good at everything, rationalise their choices. Avoid physical or emotional overload at school. Life involves opportunities and priorities. Focus on three musical instruments. Not six.

Dedicate a free night in the week and over the weekend for your family to meet, greet and eat together.

Many grounded parents consider their parental responsibilities. They get the work and life balance right. I respect their parenting. So will their children one day.

An elite subset of parents embrace the commitments of extra-curricular activities because their child is passionate and talented in a specific pursuit. These are the parents whose child will swim, row, sail, run or play for Australia at the Olympic Games or international sporting meets. They believe and support their child's dream to write, act, sing, perform, invent or create. There must be a place reserved for facilitating the giftedness of our artistic, athletic and scientific students. They provide an intellectual and emotional cohesiveness that forms the basis of a civilised society and ensures our humanity.

Take the busy out of life

Parents are pressured to outsource their parenting to entertain children. They should be confident to allow children to use their own imagination and play. Children need time to think, create, play, self-direct and be happy. With these skills, children learn how to self-regulate and be still.

It can be difficult to maintain a calm household when parents are doing shift work or high-pressured jobs with long hours. Western Australia has a strong mining culture which pays well. It demands fly-in fly-out (FIFO) rosters. These can be antisocial for families and detrimental to the mental health of vulnerable workers. Nursing and medical rosters can also be disruptive to the routine of young families.

In busy households, particularly when both parents work, electronic devices can become proxy child minders and tools for lazy learning. Children lack the benefit from consistent rules and firm but fair boundaries implemented by parents. This makes them anxious and insecure.

Less can be more within some homes. Many people embrace a simple lifestyle. They opt out of conventional lifestyle choices. Some families elect a period of home schooling as an effective 'time-out' from the pressures of mainstream education. This can assist their struggling child to learn the basic core learning areas of numeracy and literacy.

Other families have literally packed up their home and grown together by connecting with the land and travelling around our beautiful country.

Connectivity with nature can provide nurture and peace for our minds and bodies. Planned travel can create creative and reflective thinking time for children. It teaches them the value and meaning of time. They experience the myriad shades of the day which they can't experience from their covered classroom.

My mother constantly writes and tells me to 'take time to smell the flowers'. Of course I never do! I tell her that the time to do that is death. But, as someone who has parented in the fast lane, I strongly advise you to spend time in the slow lane. This will give you the opportunity to watch and enjoy your child grow.

The social shift which encompasses the way we connect with nature and each other threatens to impact on our mental and physical health. Spend time during your pregnancy reconnecting with nature, friends, family and yourself. You are then ready to connect with your baby from birth. This will help you relate better later with your pre-teen and teenager.

Fast-forwarding childhood

Children of 10 years of age want to be 15. First, they need to have a go at 'being 10'. Our society needs to be better at acknowledging the tween years and helping children secure a strong sense of self during this time. This protects them from developing a personality disorder in early adult life.

There is no smooth transition across the pre-adolescent years. Parents who plan for the bumps will come out less shattered. Consistent parenting, being calm in the midst of chaos, reflective decisions and selflessness will help weather these tumultuous years. Parental love is about sacrificing or deferring personal aims to focus on the important job of raising a child.

Parents that I speak with indicate that parenting is hard when children are little. Parenting becomes even harder as children grow. The physical hard work of parenting is replaced with the more emotionally demanding task of mentoring a recalcitrant teenager. You love them to bits, but there will be times when you dislike them immensely.

For some families, the structure, safety nets and stability of the early childhood years can unexpectedly change. This happens when there is an illness or death in the family, a beloved family pet dies, a parent loses their job or there is a change in home or school location. The genetically or environmentally vulnerable child is emotionally derailed if they are a victim to an adverse childhood event. This can result from parental separation, the escalation of brewing sibling rivalry or emotional, physical or sexual abuse.

The impact of mental distress

The mental distress and addiction of a child or parent can shatter family units. It becomes a long-term burden spread over extended family and community. Disorders implicated include depression, suicide, anxiety, self-harm, eating disorders, adjustment disorders, personality disorders, mood disorders, bipolar disorders and schizophrenia.

Children diagnosed with ADHD, autism and significant learning disabilities can carry the comorbidity of some of these mental illnesses. This makes parenting even harder.

Mental distress may present for the first time during the formative years from 10 to 15 years. Children with autism, severe anxiety, depression or poor body self-image struggle with the physical, emotional and social transition which occurs from Year 5 to Year 10 at school. This coincides with the shift from primary to high school.

These are the vulnerable 'red flag' years. Parents must remain vigilant and read the subtle signs of the child who becomes depressed through stealth. It is a bit like watching a child drown. Children drown silently. Depressed children can die under our watch. They conceal their depression. We misread the signs of their altered mood as normal teenage aloofness, grunge dressing, late nights and antisocial behaviours.

Parents have to focus on emotional and social resilience during these years and ignore school grades. The anxious or depressed student will disengage from education. A happy and confident child is well placed to perform academically. School marks are not important until about Year 10 when grades determine subject options and future academic choices.

Your child won't fall too far behind academically if you focus on numeracy and literacy early. Your child needs to develop a sense of belonging, and a love and incentive for learning and the pursuit of a passion. This is the best way for them to engage with school and further education. They can't do this if they are sad, stressed or lonely.

Childhood SPECS from 10 to 15 years

Social and emotional
Social skills and emotional resilience are the most important milestones to focus on during pre-adolescence and the teenage years. These competencies determine your child's academic performance more than intellectual ability.

Acknowledge your teenager's growing independence. Respect it – stand back, shut up and listen. Be there to help when they need you.

Adolescence shouldn't be about you. It is about your emerging adult. If you aren't coping with this developmental phase, they won't. Seek professional advice for yourself and for them.

Speech and language
Many children outgrow or largely overcome early language problems. Most children respond to timely speech intervention for a lisp or stutter and by now have overcome early articulation problems. Stuttering or dysfluent speech can run in families and affects boys more than girls. It can recur and responds to a positive and supportive parenting approach, with speech pathology guidance.

Adolescents with high functioning autism, typically of Asperger type, may speak in an odd way. They adopt an accent or unusual intonation. Depressed kids sound 'flat' and have a monotonous quality to their voice.

Language difficulties can be linked with a subtle learning problem or meet the criteria of dyslexia or dysgraphia – specific learning disorders that have previously been discussed.

Students with high functioning autism often have an extensive vocabulary. Their writing has great humour and creativity but with literal, concrete and, at times, rigid and repetitive content. Bright students with HFA can rote learn thousands of words and learn multiple social scenarios to fit in with their peer group. If you challenge them with complex language concepts, they become quite stressed. They learn that 'huge' means 'big', but argue with you when you suggest that 'huge' can also mean 'intense', 'mammoth', 'significant' or 'life-changing'.

Children with diagnosed inattentive ADHD and language-based learning problems classically present with problems in initiating and completing written work. They find it hard to get ideas down on paper, especially when there is a time pressure. Orally, they excel and are innovative visual learners. This is not always acknowledged.

Physicality

Kids need a strength to take with them to high school. This helps them transition when they commence Year 7 at around 12 years of age.

Physicality, especially for boys attending a single gender school, is important. Physical limitations can affect general fitness levels, motivation and gross motor and fine motor coordination skills. They have a significant impact on children during the early high school years – socially, emotionally and academically.

Children with ADHD, anxiety, autism, hypermobility and developmental coordination disorder (dyspraxia) can be clumsy.

High school can be an unhappy place for them if they don't attend the school that best suits their emotional needs. This means being lucky with the mix of students, parents and teachers in your child's year.

If this is a bad mix, you have to work out ways to survive, grow and flourish. If this is not possible, after every effort has been made by yourself and the school, you have to consider moving your child. This is a big decision with ramifications. It deserves much reflection and even professional input. It is one of those decisions best slept upon.

Physical competency is glorified in some schools. It is applauded in the same way as some schools parade their academic success. Physical or academic prowess can be celebrated, but not at the expense of belittling the role of the normal student.

Forcing poor swimmers to enter a novelty race during their high school years because they aren't fast enough to compete can be demeaning. If they are not good enough, they know that, and are probably quite happy to cheer their colleagues on from the sidelines. Novelty swimming races in high school are like getting a participation ribbon. They don't make sense. Most children will ultimately do best when they have a sense of belonging.

Fatigue syndromes

Very anxious children can be physically immobilised by their anxiety. They can have overwhelming fatigue. It can be impossible for them to pick up a pen or pencil.

A prior physical or mental illness can precipitate a severe chronic fatigue condition. Classically, viral infections such as glandular fever precipitate this complex condition. Elite athletes have succumbed to the devastation of physical exhaustion over time spans exceeding twelve months, before regaining their physical fitness.

Children with autism and ADHD can have hypermobility of their joints which makes them tire and fatigue readily. They can suffer with chronic fatigue symptoms, especially if subjected to academic or sporting performance anxiety.

Children with debilitating fatigue become removed from their peers due to limited school attendance. They are at greater risk of being targeted for bullying, including social exclusion.

Social media engagement can be helpful for these kids to keep them in the social loop when they are not going to school. These students will require close school liaison and a modified physical attendance school program to keep them engaged with education. Once students are in the final school years, it becomes more difficult for those with mental health and physical needs to meet the demands of the education curriculum.

Depression

Children and adolescents with severe depression can be 'frozen' by physical incapacity. This further isolates them from school and their peer group and perpetuates a cycle of greater social isolation and depression. Their fitness is compromised. Sleeping and eating patterns are disturbed.

Eating disorders and depression are complex mental health disorders which afflict students in the high school years. They lead to social and academic withdrawal. Severe clinical cases require inpatient medical management.

Ongoing liaison with school, healthcare professionals and families, special consideration for assessments and external exams, and individually tailored school programs will be necessary. This may include special permission to complete high school over thirteen years and a protracted tertiary program with alternative pathway entry.

Down syndrome

Children with Down syndrome can have instability of their upper cervical spine. This makes it dangerous for them to do horse riding or contact sports such as football or rugby. An X-ray or MRI of their spine will exclude this anomaly.

Heart problems

Some families have unusual cardiac problems which increase the risk of sudden death. Seek an opinion from a cardiologist if your child wants to play elite sport and there is a significant family history of cardiac problems. This includes a history of heart attack under the age of 40 years.

Periodically, we hear the tragic news of the young athlete who kicks a goal, then collapses and dies on the football or rugby field. There is no logic or sense for these random events.

School avoidance and non-attendance

Social and academic withdrawal is prevalent in teenage children with anxiety and with high functioning autism. It is a significant problem and is emerging as one of the hardest mental health problems to deal with, together with disordered eating patterns and eating disorders.

The age group 10 to 15 years is the most vulnerable but least supported within our health and mental health systems. Any family who has tried to obtain help for their 14- or 15-year-old child who refuses to attend school and medical or psychology appointments, or is anxious, depressed and emotionally dysregulated, will attest to this.

Anxiety

Anxiety is the single most salient cause of school disengagement, academic under-performance and school dropout. It amplifies the problems of teenagers with autism, many of whom appear to regress for a period during adolescence.

Sad and anxious teenagers can end up staying at home. If their families and healthcare professionals are not supportive, patient, tolerant and gently encouraging, they can become socially withdrawn and reclusive in adult life.

To prevent this very negative outcome you must seek help early for the child who is anxious upon high school entry. The added expectation of social and academic performance in a large and new high school environment compounds the social and generalised anxiety in a vulnerable child.

High functioning autism

All children experience anxiety with change. This can be over-whelming in the child with high functioning autism and place them in a static state. Unless you have witnessed this, you cannot comprehend the impact of debilitating childhood anxiety.

Schools and teachers have great insight into this problem and deal with it compassionately. But, some teachers and bystanders don't understand the concept of severe anxiety in children. They label them as manipulative or lazy.

Hopefully, with education and greater public awareness of emotional and physical illness, this misconception will shift.

Anxiety can lead to depression in adolescence. In puberty it can present as social and cognitive regression. We often miss depression in children with autism.

A 13-year-old boy with autism gave me a wonderful insight into how it feels to have a brain that can get angry and sad. He had a great teacher, who asked for his input in making up his Individual Education Plan (IEP). He recognised when he was getting upset and asked that people talk softly and calmly to him when he started to get angry. This helped him settle down. When he was really agitated he said he needed everyone to back off and leave him alone. This worked for him and his teacher.

He also developed a coloured-card system which he used to grade his level of anxiety. This allowed him to convey in a visual format how he was feeling.

The bright, high-functioning child with autism, the child with ADHD and anxiety, or the gifted student shackled by anxiety and perfectionism have significant disabilities. The school system demands constant timed assessments for the final three years of high school. This places extreme and unfair pressure on students who frequently disengage from the education process. Attempts to re-engage students by insisting that they hand in written work within the structure of a formal or virtual classroom underestimates the enormity of the burden that timed assessments place on them.

Whilst our high school and tertiary education systems provide many varied and flexible pathways, there will always remain a small cohort of very capable students whom we fail as parents, medical professionals and educators. These often include children with high functioning autism, especially those in whom the diagnosis is missed. These children do better when a diagnosis of autism spectrum disorder is made during their early school years.

Home schooling

Some children with autism can't cope with the social pressures of school, even when safety nets and structure are provided. Some parents are then faced with home-based education which can work well. But, it doesn't solve the long-term problem of successfully assimilating a socially anxious child into the wider community.

Parents feel isolated and abandoned when leaving the intensity of a school structure to the more relaxed boundaries of home education. Parents who home school their children receive support from caring and experienced home education moderators. Parents who home school a child with autism require even greater assistance.

School phobia

Home schooling or online government-supported distant education may be required for the anxious child who can't face their fears or attend school. They are not school 'refusers'. These kids can't physically or emotionally face the school environment. They have school phobia and are emotionally traumatised by anything pertaining to school. Even the sight of a school uniform can make them feel physically sick.

Significant anxiety and school avoidance are best understood as a form of post-traumatic stress. When it occurs you have to back off from any school obligations until a student is well enough emotionally to re-engage with learning on their terms. This may not happen until they are a mature-aged student of 20 or older.

Focus on encouraging them to have an interest – music, media, art, cooking, woodcraft, design and textiles or technology. You want them to think and to use their brains.

Structure is important. An anxious child needs some scaffolding and goals, even if minor. This gives them a sense of purpose and success. Initially this may be as simple as a regular bedtime, bath time and mealtime.

Try to have one external goal outside the home each day, so that a child doesn't retreat into the safety of their home or room. This can lead to the socially restricting condition of agoraphobia, an irrational fear of public places.

Intensive therapy with a competent and experienced clinical psychologist is warranted. Weekly sessions are time-consuming and expensive, but can be necessary.

Medication includes the judicious and monitored use of drugs. Selective serotonin reuptake inhibitors (SSRIs) such as sertraline and fluoxetine can be helpful. An atypical antipsychotic such as risperidone or aripiprazole may be part of treatment. Both drugs need regular clinical input from a paediatrician, psychiatrist or both.

Physically or emotionally forcing an adolescent child to attend school once they have disengaged from learning is like force-feeding a young child with food anxiety or food phobia. There is no place for physically dragging the anxious, avoidant student to school against their will.

The more you push a child who is anxious and emotionally compromised, the more likely that child will oppose your efforts. They will externalise their anxiety by directing their verbal and physical anger towards you as a parent or a teacher. Or, they become a 'tortoise' and retreat into a shell of avoidance and depression.

Parents need to combat anxiety in early childhood by taking charge without being controlling. This is their best chance to modify the path of childhood anxiety which can lead to avoidant behaviours. They need to act when a child first presents with anxiety and seek professional help.

School choices

In Australia we have great schools in the government and private sector. This provides choice for families and their children. Decisions about schooling should be made on the emotional and social fit of the school and student and not on academic results alone.

If a child is happy and emotionally secure they can optimise their cognitive potential. If they are at a school where they are relentlessly bullied, or the academic and social pressure is too great, they will fail.

Once you decide which school to send your child to, stick to your decision. Avoid transferring your child on the grounds of academic progress if they are socially happy and enjoy school.

I am grateful to my parents for moving me from the local high school I attended after we relocated from a small NSW town to Melbourne. I remember walking into one of the Year 7 classrooms. There was no academic challenge. I was victimised and socially bullied. Three weeks later I was walking into a much smaller and traditional-style classroom at a private girls' school. I could tell that learning was encouraged in that classroom. That was the first day I came home from high school happy.

You must listen to your child.

The curse of giftedness

Intellectually and gifted students should be given the opportunity to pursue their giftedness in a holistic way. Selective schools assess children as young as 10 years old on discrete parameters such as intellect, music, visual arts or drama. Most gifted students achieve in all academic areas. They may also be musical, dramatic or athletic. Others are 'doubly gifted'. This means they are advanced in maths, but have a specific learning disorder such as dyslexia.

Some students with high functioning autism have a discrete area of high intelligence, often in technology, maths or the arts. But, they have a low social and emotional intelligence quotient (IQ). It is hard for them to cope with th transition to high school with its high social and academic expectations.

Schools dedicated to the specific needs of academically gifted children must maintain a balance in their academic program. When this happens, bright students succeed. This doesn't always happen. Focusing on science, without promoting the arts, won't produce the best innovators, inventors and creators. We have to get children to utilise their whole brain capacity.

Paediatric and education liaison

Paediatricians are not educators. We are not trained to teach, nor are we competent in pedagogy. We have limited liaison with the teachers, counsellors and psychologists that are entrusted with the education and care of our children. Yet, paediatricians and psychiatrists are asked to provide expert opinion that will influence and determine the type of education a child receives.

Paediatricians evaluate children to determine whether they are eligible to receive extra assistance within classrooms, or have access to dedicated education support facilities. They advocate for a student to receive additional time in examinations for a number of learning disorders, including dyslexia and dysgraphia.

It is insulting for an experienced educator to be told by a paediatrician which student in their class requires extra education assistance. Educators are best placed to determine this and decide where extra input is necessary.

An 'elastic' education system would stretch to cater for all children. It would be needs-based, rather than one which allocates funds for diagnosed disability. Assigning an education assistant or second teacher to every primary school classroom, at least during the first five years from kindergarten to Year 3, is logical and probably financially efficient. The teacher would then have a support person within the class at all times, important for mentorship and protective for the teacher should there be allegations of teacher misconduct. This would particularly be helpful for those students with learning disorders who later enter the high school system.

Teach more, test less

We stifle a child's desire to learn when we constantly test what they don't know. Students avoid hard subjects such as maths if they fear getting a poor mark which can affect their school graduation score. Student anxiety results from the performance pressure they are under during their latter high school years. This contributes to teacher anxiety.

If we can't teach a cohort of predominantly 'normal ability' students over the course of fourteen years and give them a robust education, we have a flawed system.

There is concern about Australia's falling rankings on OECD (Organisation for Economic Co-operation and Development) education tables and poor adult literacy. If this trend continues, universities and other tertiary institutions will be forced to implement their own entry examinations. They are likely to insist on prerequisite subjects for defined professions so that students are not academically naïve and destined for failure.

Educators talk about a greater focus on STEM subjects. These are *Science, Technology, Engineering* and *Mathematics*. The emphasis during the school years needs to be on STEMS, or *Social skills, Technology, English, Mathematics* and *Science.*

Children who can socialise, empathise, communicate and problem-solve have the tools to learn, to innovate and create. We need to rethink the philosophy of how we educate our children. This dictates that we revise the way parents raise their children.

Social rips

The tides of change

Working at the coalface I get a preview of social change. Families have increased financial hardship. Kids are saying that mum or dad are worried and that mum is crying because they don't have enough money. Families are downsizing their home to increase equity and families are splitting up under the strain. This fuels parental and childhood anxiety and is having an impact on family life.

Parents try to get extra work. Higher-paid FIFO jobs take working mothers away from their partner and children and give them the role of being the main breadwinner. Many fathers can't cope with this responsibility, as they don't get treated as equals with women in the child-rearing race. Some leave the parental partnership, especially if there is the added burden of a child with an intellectual disability, autism or mental distress. But, a lot of dads stay. They need support and encouragement in their difficult parental role.

Private school enrolments are slowing as more parents choose well-performing public schools for their child's education.

Some of my obstetric colleagues say they have fewer private bookings because of the financial worries of families.

Life will become less busy because families won't be able to afford the cost of organised extracurricular activities for their children. They will have to opt for family outings to their local park and play board, video and card games on the weekends with their kids. This is not a bad thing.

Dependent on the strength of the Australian dollar and stock market volatility, families will swap international holidays for holidays at home. The heightened global terrorist threat is part of our future. It impacts on family decisions.

Social gaps

Our social climate has significantly altered and has an impact on the health and mental health of children.

A young mother asked me when she should have started to clean her child's teeth, after they had become seriously decayed. She thought that you waited until the baby teeth fell out because the first teeth were only temporary.

Basic parenting is not intuitive for some families. A broadening gap exists between families with means and those who struggle financially. The gap is not just about annual household income or racial background. It is about the families that have access to technology and education and a stable living environment and those that don't.

When I read about houses blowing up because of a home methamphetamine (ice) lab exploding, I think of the emotional, social and physical deprivation endured by the children within those environments. The pervasiveness of drug addiction in our families and communities is a shared responsibility, because it affects all of us.

Children from privileged homes are referred to as having been 'born with a silver spoon' in their mouths. That exclusivity doesn't always protect them from adversity.

Addictive behaviour starts young – even at school. Methamphetamine use crosses all social boundaries and destroys us all. The pervasiveness of addiction is best tackled as a health and mental health issue. It is not just a law and order problem.

Narcissism and self-harm in the teenage years

Trapped in the mirror

A generation of overpraise in children has contributed to narcissistic traits in the teenage years. This social flaw is captured by the 'selfie'.

Narcissism has a significant impact on adolescents and their parents. Kids seek their few seconds of fame online. Earlier generations fainted at the sight of The Beatles, Madonna or Elton John. The difference is that kids are now obsessed by fame. It is important for teenagers to have passion, but they risk losing their own self-identity through the desperate pursuit of someone else's fame. Kids set themselves up for failure by aspiring to unrealistic dreams.

Internet access enables the emotionally naïve and socially immature adolescent to post digital images of themselves. These are permanent digital markers and subject to cyberbullying attacks, exposure to sex predators and hacking practices such as doxxing.

Impulsive social media engagement by adolescents is extremely difficult for 'techno-dinosaur' parents to monitor. Parents have to educate themselves about navigating social media. They must actively manage the use of electronic devices and instil healthy habits of electronic exposure in their children. This has to be done early.

Self-harm

The ambitious teenager who posts their greatest photo or song on Facebook or YouTube is exposing themselves to the public domain. When they are disliked and the target of cyberbullying and internet trolls they become depressed, anxious and angry. They feel hopeless, hate their life and start to self-harm by cutting. Dangerous conversations on social media occur in the early hours of the morning with drunk or depressed participants.

The vulnerable teenager tries to gain sympathy by participating in the teenage cult of disillusionment and self-harm. Online sites show kids ways to do this, such as the ice and salt challenge. This causes caustic burns to skin and can require skin grafts.

High school students participate in 'concealed cutting'. This self-harm consists of serial cuts made to the skin of the upper thigh with visual images posted on Facebook.

Older teenagers engage in the 'emoji' challenge. They burn their skin with the tip of a lighter, leaving the markings of a smiley face.

A Year 8 student described her distress at confronting peers in the toilet block at her local high school engaging in erotic asphyxiation behaviours. The alleged approach by the school was to lock up the girls' toilets. She told her family she couldn't stay at her school.

Schools need more support
Schools have to deal with the cult of overt and covert cutting and other self-harm practices. These dysfunctional behaviours are an

epidemic amongst teenage girls in Years 8, 9 and 10. They need confrontation, not cover up.

High schools need more psychologists, not security guards. The management of mental health is too complex to place on the caseload of burdened teachers. If your child is cutting, seek professional help with a doctor, clinical psychologist, paediatrician and sometimes a psychiatrist.

Younger children who scratch, gouge or pinch their skin, pluck their eyelashes or even bite their nails are demonstrating early signs of self-harm. A psychologist helps a young person develop strategies to deal with the feelings of anxiety, low self-esteem and emotional dysregulation which can lead to self-harm. Impulsivity associated with hyperactive ADHD contributes to these behaviours.

Our high schools have significant cohorts of young Year 9 and 10 students who seek notoriety with fellow students who cut, starve, binge and drink. Or, try unprotected and risky sex or designer drugs. Most Year 9 and 10 students have some experience or awareness of the use of marijuana (cannabis). Some have heard about NBOMe, a relatively new drug, implicated in the deaths of several Australian high school students. Its use is facilitated by the ease of passage by post, embedded in flat wafers which can be ingested.

Year 10 is a dangerous drug year. It is the year when parties, sleepovers, bodies and vodka are shared.

A 13-year-old high school student told me, 'We have lots of drugs, alcohol and sex in our high school'. He had already worked out that he was safest as a nerd. This student made the mature decision to affiliate himself with a social group perceived as inferior to what he described as 'the jocks' and 'stoners'.

If your child attends a public government high school, you may not get a parent contact list. Attend any coffee mornings or parent nights that are arranged independently from the school. This gives you an opportunity to get some contact numbers and local class knowledge. When your child attends sleepovers and class parties it helps to have some reliable parent details. Private schools have a more formal process for assisting families to assimilate class lists in which you are included, unless you opt out.

Stay put

Be the smoke detector

Your kids need you more in the pre-teen and teenage years, than when they were crawling around in nappies or still tripping and falling. You must be the lurking shadow in the background. The sense of you has to be around.

Avoid complacency when reaching significant milestones such as your child turning double-digits in age. Any small flaws in your parenting, your child's self-identity or family dynamics can become giant clefts during the pre-adolescent and adolescent years. Small problems, which seemed inconsequential during the busyness of the early primary school years, suddenly appear daunting and overwhelming.

Don't catastrophise the petty problems. Take time to talk with your partner. Engage in self-talk and personal reflection. Try 'mindfulness' or 'heartfulness'.

Work out parenting strategies when you are calm. Don't be the 'panic parent' who overreacts or makes impulsive or explosive decisions about life events during stressful times. This is pertinent when choosing schools and extracurricular activities. These are the things most likely to define your child. Whilst sometimes the worst thing to do is nothing, a well-timed pause can be helpful.

Early adolescence is a time when peers and others have more influence on your child than a parent. You hope your conversations, love and patience have been sufficiently nurturing for your child to trust and come to you for support and guidance. This may be about bullying at school, feeling sad, or homework problems. You need to be accessible to your children during this difficult transition.

Puberty happens

Sex and Stuff

Most parents are grateful that schools manage sex education. Talking to your growing child about the pubertal changes of their body should be straightforward, but it isn't. When your child bravely asks you a question about sex, answer it promptly, simply and honestly. Don't ask the question, 'Why?' If your child wants to know something about sex, they just do, so tell them. Give an honest but age-appropriate answer.

Assign female and male body parts their correct anatomical names. A penis isn't a person, so it doesn't warrant being given a name. There are excellent books with simple illustrations that you can read or give your child. They help a child work out what life is all about. Resist the temptation to fast-forward the sex education syllabus in one sitting to get it out of the way. If your child has heard enough, stop. There are times to talk about topics such as sexually transmitted infections. This may not be when talking with your 10-year-old child.

Conversations about sex can be an opportunity to talk about good and bad touching and sexual privacy. If your child makes a sexual disclosure to you as their parent or other responsible adult, believe them and seek professional help.

Fathers need to be aware that pubertal changes occur in girls as early as 8 and 9 years of age. Some fathers who attend medical appointments with their 10- or 11-year-old daughter have clearly not recognised that their daughter is changing. They still treat them as if they were the cute little girl of 4 or 5.

The pre-teen requires greater physical space from a caring parent, particularly in public. Kids of this age don't enjoy their shoulders being rubbed, or hugs and shoulder nudges while they are walking through a shopping centre. They detest the sloppy, enthusiastic kiss from a relative that is forced upon them against their will.

Teenage girls like fun books such as *Girl Stuff – Your Full-On Guide to the Teen Years* by Kaz Cooke. Parents find it helpful to do some research and choose a resource for pre-adolescents to guide them through the growing years. Kids won't listen or believe what you think or say as a parent until they're in their twenties. This is too late to wait for balanced and accurate life information. Avoid your child having only peers and the internet as their moral compass during the teen years. They already have access to inappropriate social media sites which promote self-harm, glamorise eating disorders and immortalise narcissism.

Humour can help when discussing sex with your teenager.

A mother told me that her 12-year-old daughter came home from school and said that she had something to tell her. The mother was suddenly fearful that something inappropriate had occurred at school. Her daughter then stated, 'I have had my period'. When trying to think of the best response, her daughter started laughing and said, 'Just joking, I wanted to see how you would respond!' The school had discussed sexual health that day.

Talk with your teenager

Trust

The pre-adolescent child considers trust as the most important value during their developmental journey. Kids tell me of their sense of betrayal when an adult, especially a parent or teacher, lies to them or discusses and shares knowledge of their personal problems.

The disclosure of private information requires the student's consent as they approach adulthood. This is generally accepted within schools and by professionals as around the age of 16. I think we should do this even earlier, dependent on the maturity and intelligence of the child. The formal age of medical consent varies between states and territories.

To neglect involving the teenage child about decisions which can affect their life breaches trust. It jeopardises the working relationship between the child and their parent, carer, teacher, doctor, psychologist or mentor. This is why therapists have an open disclosure policy with children and adolescents.

To form an effective therapeutic relationship, the child has to trust the therapist, whether this is a clinical psychologist, school psychologist, school chaplain, social worker or youth worker. This trust has to be unconditional or the therapist will lose the child and compound the child's perception of betrayal. With an older child this means excluding the parent from the relationship.

This can appear to be a ruthless approach for parents. They are often tightly intertwined with the emotional fabric of their child due to great complexity or adverse circumstances. These parents can feel abandoned, guilty, confused, disempowered and alone. Parents must learn to step back and trust a therapist to work with their child when that child requires emotional healing.

Parents benefit from seeking their own therapist for advocacy, understanding, therapeutic and even legal intervention.

The choice of therapist for the child is integral to their healing. This can relate to the child who has experienced adverse circumstances and is anxious or depressed. It can be relevant to the child who is bullied, socially isolated, failing at school, or has an eating disorder.

You can be unlucky and have a poor fit of therapist and child. It is important that the choice of therapist is made carefully. The therapist has to be registered, accredited and have had sufficient clinical experience to responsibly care for your child. Therapy isn't always therapeutic.

A private clinical psychologist can provide timely intervention. This will incur a monetary fee. Government subsidies for clinical psychology attendances provide some relief. Speak with your family doctor about what resources and funding are available for your child.

Excellent help is also available in the public sector but waiting times tend to be longer and staff turnover greater. This can make the establishment of a long-term therapeutic relationship more difficult.

If you are struggling financially don't be afraid to speak with family. They may want to assist you – emotionally or financially. Money and time commitment spent early is a good investment for your child. It can change a child's life path. When children and adolescents need help, most parents 'move mountains' to get that help for their child. I am humbled by the resolve of the parents of a child in need.

Betrayal

Children who have been robbed of their childhood by mental distress or addiction afflicting their mother or father can take a long time to find trust in another person or relationship. Most children will stay loyal to a parent, even if this places them in a potentially damaging emotional, social or physical situation. This may occur when a parent uses alcohol or illicit drugs such as ice (crystal meth) to treat their depression.

Older children find the chaos of their dysfunctional home safer and preferable to the risks and uncertainty of a foster home. These kids grow up fast. They have to face the betrayal of a parent who lies about their drug or alcohol dependency, compliance with prescribed medication or medical appointments. This is a form of ongoing emotional abuse. Often these kids are forced to assume the parenting role within the home.

Addiction

Children and teenagers at risk need access to good mental health services. Because of the stringent intake criteria of many of these services and the high cost of private mental health services, families can be left to fend for themselves. Whilst therapeutic intervention continues to be withheld for those addicted to alcohol or drugs until they seek voluntary rehabilitation, our society will continue to fail the children of addiction.

Many hidden families, some cloaked by the respectability of middle or upper class, deal with the adversity of mental distress and addiction. Children from 10 to 15 years, or even younger, have their childhood stolen. They are hurled into proxy parenting roles because a mother or father struggling with depression or addiction is unable to cook, clean or care for them. Extended family support becomes strained under these circumstances.

Teenagers find themselves responsible for the care of younger children. They have to seek part-time work to supplement the family income. They quit school or defer their studies. Welfare agencies give up on them because of under-resourcing, lack of awareness or because a parent does not meet the bureaucratic intake criteria for their services.

If a parent has a terminal illness, society has a defined and accepted role. Community will come together and assist battling families. They will make meals, deliver children to and from school and undertake household chores such as cleaning and collecting groceries. It is harder for community to intercede when a household is shrouded in the obscurity of mental distress, heralded by screaming matches and frequent police or emergency service call-outs.

Neighbours and community don't like to interfere or get involved when social boundaries are blurred by mental health problems. Yet, physical disability is seen as a safe and concrete problem which most people feel equipped to confront. Some families have told me that they would prefer their child or partner to have a terminal illness rather than a psychologically debilitating illness.

The teenager caring for a parent with mental distress can find it very difficult to access financial, practical and sustainable assistance. They are emotionally blackmailed and sabotaged by a parent and forced to stay within a dysfunctional home. Some parents steal from the financial accounts of their children to service their own addiction, whether of alcohol, tobacco or drugs such as methamphetamine.

In the US there are specific trust accounts set up for minors or children at risk of having their childhood earnings fleeced by a parent or guardian within the entertainment industry. These are known as Coogan Accounts. Children who are captive within a dysfunctional household should have access to a similar trust account into which government welfare payments are deposited.

Speak silently to your teenager

Silence can be helpful when caught in the tirade of an angry teenager.

> *A mother gave me a good life lesson one day about how teenagers think. She had always tried to protect and rescue her adolescent from whatever difficulties were overwhelming their life. One day her daughter told her, 'Mum, it's all right, I just want to rant and I need you to listen and not say anything'.*

I have learned a lot about parenting from listening to families. It is best to do this in silence. To parent better, you have to learn humility, to listen more and speak less. Some over-protective parents find it impossible to cease nagging their teenager.

If you have not yet had children, the thought of a teenager sulking about in your home probably seems as remote as man landing on Mars. That moment comes upon you in a rush. While you still have time to conceptualise life with a child, adolescent and emerging adult, take time to ponder and reflect about your future life with them.

Most mothers will tell you that they find raising 13- to 15-year-old girls a diabolical task. They fantasise about placing their teenager in suspended animation for five years. The body language and dialogue between some teenagers and parents makes me think that the parent should be the one in 'time-out'. They would then wake up refreshed and be ready to greet their adult child.

Fault is a shared frailty. Parents and teenagers have lots of hard work to face during the transitional years from childhood to adult life. This is a time when puberty gets in the way of logic. Emotional and social issues drive the actions of your teenager. Parents need to stay on the sidelines but stay alert, ready to listen, help and take charge and act when appropriate.

There is no easy childhood phase. The 10-year-old child who tries to be the teenager before they are emotionally ready can struggle with their sense of self and be prone to anxiety or depression. A child can access adult media and aspire to dress like a teenager as soon as they reach double-digits. It is important to pace your child through these 'yearning years'.

When you have your own child you will work out your priorities and preferential parenting strategies. You will frequently get things wrong and have to revise your parenting plans. One way to get things almost right is to get the best balance between work and leisure for your family. You can't defer the duties of parenthood. This commitment will take time and will involve you stumbling and bumbling your way through the early childhood years. This challenge is called parenting.

Eating disorders

Reluctant friends

Anxiety, ADHD, SLD and ASD are joined by eating disorders during the pre-teen and teen years. Gender and demographics can't fend off this foe. It is important that you are knowledgeable about this condition to prevent it taking hold of your child and family. The mental health impact of this disorder is significant.

Anorexia nervosa and bulimia

Eating disorders are identified by the labels anorexia nervosa (AN) and less often bulimia nervosa (BN). They occur when persistent restriction of calories results in an unhealthy weight range and can be accompanied by obsessive exercise. Binge eating is characterised by periods of uncontrolled excess eating and can be followed by induced vomiting or diuretic and laxative abuse. It may not result in weight loss. These conditions affect all genders, ages and life stages.

The media is blamed for potent visual imagery which focuses on the appearance and thinness of models and actors. Eating disorders constitute a complex and convoluted spectrum. Their notoriety feeds off the frenzy of sensationalism they promote. There is the misconception that eating disorders occur only in vulnerable teenage girls. This cohort is stereotyped as the bright, high-achieving, anxious kids, fighting for control and a sense of self within households that are controlling, rigid and socially and academically pushy.

Eating disorders are pervasive. They cross all socio-economic, gender, age and parenting boundaries. Eating disorders and associated mental health conditions can run in families or occur de novo. The role of genetics is actively being considered in the aetiology of these conditions.

The diagnosis and treatment of eating disorders is an extremely difficult clinical area and outside the realm of this book to fully detail. I discuss it to increase awareness of how it presents. It is important for the mental health of your child and family that you recognise the early signs of an eating disorder and seek professional intervention. This can prevent the sequelae of chronic eating disorders and the comorbidity of depression, anxiety and borderline personality disorder.

In Australia, the National Eating Disorders Collaboration describes four types of eating disorders recognised under the *DSM-5*. These are anorexia nervosa (AN), bulimia nervosa (BN), binge eating disorder (BED) and other specified feeding and eating disorders (OSFED). The high morbidity and mortality of eating disorders is due to the detrimental physical and mental health consequences of an entrenched eating disorder. They affect about 1 in 20 Australians.

Research documents an increased risk of mortality and suicidality of these disorders when compared with the normal population. Individuals with anorexia nervosa are reported to have the highest rates, with around 1 in 5 deaths from anorexia nervosa being due to suicide. This is a disturbing figure in the context of an increasing rate of eating disorders in our country.

As a paediatrician I see many children across all developmental stages with an atypical approach to food. I am not saying that the young child who refuses to eat broccoli or fruit will develop an eating disorder. But, we have created significant social anxiety about food. This reflects the way we raise our children.

Early disordered eating patterns

Toddlers around 18 months to 2 years of age often develop selective eating habits. Parents struggle to commit to a balanced diet which includes fruit, vegetables, cereals and grains, dairy and red meat, chicken and fish. Out of desperation, some parents introduce a high-fat, high-sugar diet with a predominance for dairy. This promotes obesity and iron deficiency in children and leads to bad eating patterns in older children. Teenagers are notorious for adopting poor and erratic eating habits.

Children with autism can limit their food choices because of sensory problems and fixations. This is often problematic during the toddler years and continues throughout childhood. Forcing these children to eat food outside their comfort zone can increase their fear of food. The introduction of new foods has to be done very slowly.

Therapists such as occupational therapists and psychologists can assist this process by using a number of techniques, including social stories and sensory techniques. They can apply a behavioural approach to teach children with autism to eat a wider range of foods. Parents and families have an active role in making meal times a family routine. The focus of food within homes should be about social connectivity and not about the food.

Supplementing the diet in anxious and food-avoidant children can be stressful and result in unhelpful battles over food. Autistic, very anxious and obsessive children can develop fixed food routines. This leads to supermarket-hopping in an endeavour to source the particular brand of vanilla yoghurt or breakfast cereal that a child will eat. Discontinuation of a branded food staple can cause enormous stress within these households.

Weight focus

Young boys and girls between the ages of 5 to 10 years express concerns about their weight. Parents and doctors dismiss these comments as trivial. They don't adequately consider the vulnerabilities of the child.

Some children have a low body mass index (BMI). Their weight is much less compared with their height. It can be normal for children to follow a low growth centile. This can be seen in children with a familial and genetic predisposition to being thin and in children with certain medical conditions. The very young child with a low BMI can also present with an early disordered eating pattern.

It is the attitude to food, exercise and social routine within the household that is important to consider when assessing an underweight child. It is important to look at growth curves over time and exclude sudden or rapid weight loss. Some childhood medications can be associated with appetite suppression and weight loss such as the stimulants methylphenidate and dexamphetamine. So can medical conditions like acute diabetes.

Doctors should exclude medical causes for poor weight gain such as thyroid conditions, coeliac disease due to a gluten intolerance or gut malabsorption.

Turning vegetarian

Markers for early disordered eating patterns occur in young children of both sexes. The primary school child in Year 5 who tells you that their teacher or a friend's sister is vegetarian can be at risk of changing their eating habits. Children start to exclude meat from their diet and declare that they are vegetarian.

Families who are vegetarian feed their children with a healthy, balanced diet which contains iron sources and nutrients from non-animal sources. They continue to provide food sources such as dairy and eggs. Vegetarian families recognise the importance of the early growing years and the concept of informed consent when making a decision to exclude animal products from a child's diet. Many of these parents still give their children some red or white meat, including chicken or fish.

Young children who declare that they are vegetarian or vegan risk becoming iron and vitamin B12 deficient and restricting their calorie intake. The typical sequel is the child's refusal to eat fat in the form of dairy products. They start to skip meals, usually breakfast and then lunch. They develop a routine of daytime fasting and lose weight.

Diet and exercise

Dieting is recognised as a risk factor for eating disorders. It is linked with excessive weight gain. This same cohort start exercising more. This occurs in extracurricular programs which encourage dedicated training hours and healthy eating. They include formal swimming training, gymnastics, athletics and dance.

The child who jumps up and down or runs back and forth in their bedroom may be obsessively exercising. Parents have to consider the balance of their child's hyperactivity. Ensure a child isn't self-medicating their problems with physical activity in the same way that adults self-medicate with alcohol or drugs to treat depression or anxiety.

When a child starts to lose weight they get positive comments from peers about their altered body shape. Initially they feel happier and more driven. They adhere to a calorie-restricted or rigorous exercise-driven program. Food restriction becomes an obsession and then an addiction. It starts to control the child's life and that of their family. These children show a heightened interest in food and prepare varied and tasty dishes which they offer to everyone except themselves.

Concealed weight loss

Kids stock up on water, lollies and fast food. They try to hide their fading body contours behind loose clothes. Some kids water load, by drinking lots of fluid, or add heavy objects into pockets to falsify their body weight. They take laxatives to purge themselves of bad feelings related to weight gain.

Meal time

If given the opportunity in a busy household, children with disordered eating patterns avoid communal meal times. It is important to have regular sit-down family meal times. Eat sensibly and don't make a fuss about food.

Through social modelling, kids need to see that dinnertime can be a positive family experience. Would you go back to a restaurant where the waitperson was rude and the food uninviting? Why should your own child want to stay at 'your restaurant' if it was an unpleasant place to visit?

It is not the time for a significant male figure to comment on the body image of a teenage girl, or for a mother to nag their son or daughter about picking at their food or not eating enough. I often hear mothers talk in front of their pre-teen child about them having 'puppy fat' or commenting on them putting on weight in preparation for a growth spurt. This is potentially dangerous talk.

How eating disorders can present

One inappropriate comment can trigger a trajectory of abnormal eating in an emotionally, socially and genetically vulnerable kid. For one child this could be a comment about eating chocolate or ice-cream. It might stem from watching someone count the calories of a restaurant meal or dissect their food. This teaches the 'at risk' child how to manipulate food around the plate while maintaining the premise of eating.

School uniforms and teenage habits conceal the degree of weight loss from families, peers and teachers until it becomes extreme. This can occur very quickly. A child can rapidly go from being functional and productive to withdrawn, depressed, lethargic and unwell. They start fainting or feel cold all the time. Their heart rate slows and running or exercising is exhausting.

You notice the development of fine, downy hair, known as lanugo, on their arms and lower legs. Hair on their head can become dry and even fall out. More systemic physical problems can include dental problems; bone loss, known as osteoporosis; the loss of periods or amenorrhoea; memory and cognition problems; metabolic disturbances; and abnormal heart rhythms. These children are at extreme medical risk if exposed to a sub-optimal external environment such as flying at altitude or swimming in cold water.

Binge eating

Some children don't have extreme weight loss but continue to overexercise. They binge eat by consuming large volumes of food in the afternoons or during the night. They hide food or steal it from home or school. These children may take laxatives to give themselves diarrhoea or start habitual vomiting. This can herald a pattern of eating disorder known as bulimia. The family dentist can pick this up because of the shiny appearance at the back of the teeth. In the older child a dentist may not be able to disclose this finding to a parent because of privacy and confidentiality issues. Bulimia is a significant eating disorder. It can carry severe mental health comorbidity, including self-harm and suicide.

Confronting eating disorders

Outsiders often notice a child's weight loss before it becomes apparent to the family. Schools are in a delicate position to raise concerns about a very thin child. They find it difficult to approach families, especially those who hide mental health problems behind the mask of professionalism, elitism or privacy.

By the time a family realises that their child has an eating problem it can be difficult to access timely, appropriate or adequate support. Families find themselves in crisis and are forced to attend an emergency department for help. It can take several months to get an appointment to be seen in a dedicated tertiary eating disorder clinic. Even within the private sector, there is limited access to people with expertise in this area.

Access to services

In Western Australia, our tertiary teaching hospital for children cuts off their acute intake at 16 years. For the adolescent between the ages of 15 and 18 years there are limited healthcare options for the management of mental health problems such as eating disorders, particularly if hospitalisation for starvation is necessary. Adult medical or psychiatric wards are not appropriate. They don't cater for specific adolescent needs.

Many private psychologists delineate eating disorders as outside their area of expertise. This is because they are high-risk mental health disorders which carry great comorbidity. They affect the child, the family, schools and peers. Eating disorders are chronic and high maintenance. They can be particularly difficult to manage in the teenage girl with high functioning autism or depression and in the teenage boy who engages in competitive sports.

The management of eating disorders is best with a specialised tertiary team. This includes paediatric gastroenterologists, paediatricians, psychiatrists, clinical psychologists, social workers, mental health and general nurses, dieticians, physiotherapists, occupational therapists and teachers.

Early detection

The early recognition and treatment of a suspected eating disorder is a priority during the childhood and adolescent years. The role of the family doctor is pivotal in their early detection. When a young child presents to their doctor for a school medical prior to school camp there is a great opportunity to objectively plot and discuss healthy growth.

Checking weight regularly at home or school is not helpful. Comments alluding to dress or appearance, even if positive, don't help. This is important for fathers to remember. Don't comment if your teenage daughter is wearing make-up for the first time or boots instead of shoes. This observation is not required and may be harmful.

Schools and eating disorders

Schools are forced to address the negative effects of body image, promoted by 'selfies' and social media. This includes popular online sites which post pictures of 'the thigh gap' or emaciated bodies. Many schools already talk about eating disorders in their science, physical health or biology curriculum.

The mother of a 10-year-old girl told me that her daughter and some friends were shown by a fellow student how to induce vomiting by strategically placing their fingers down their throats. I can understand the alleged awkward response of the primary school teacher responsible for that cohort of girls.

Teachers require greater psychological backup so that they can focus on their job of teaching children to read, write and do maths. They shouldn't have to carry the burden of the mental health of students and families.

The emotional status of young people influences school performance and peer interactions. Schools require more help to address the adolescent issues they confront when young children exit the primary school years. Schools deal with the problems of students with anxiety, social and academic withdrawal, academic underachievement, depression, self-harm, suicide, alcohol and drug abuse, and eating disorders. Many of these illnesses present with emotionally dysregulated behaviours, including physical aggression and manipulative behaviours, and bullying, oppositional, defiant and confrontational actions.

School-based interventions are increasingly requested for students at risk or suffering from mental health problems. This necessitates significant dollars, diversification of a school's staff base and additional funded professional support.

Students with chronic eating disorders face hospitalisation which further stigmatises them. One of the best ways for teenagers to start recovering from mental distress is to become re-engaged with life by providing a structured and caring environment. This keeps them connected with peers. School provides this lifeline for some of these kids.

Sadly, we are not raising resilient kids. Schools are no longer just about education. They are increasingly about holistic student care. This is the path etched by social shift, parental disempowerment and family breakdown. The financial cost of this has resulted in the exponential rise of education, mental health and healthcare budgets.

Family and hospital-based intervention

Families can change the course of an eating disorder if they act early and with support. A number of management strategies are used to approach eating disorders. Positive parenting techniques work well with childhood behavioural problems and stuttering. They have a role in eating disorders.

The Maudsley approach or Family-Based Treatment (FBT) plan for the management of adolescents with anorexia nervosa has had some success, particularly for adolescents affected for less than three years. This program was devised by a team of professionals, including child and adolescent psychiatrists and psychologists at the Maudsley Hospital in London.

It involves an intensive outpatient schedule, using parents and siblings to take an active role and gradually hand back the control of food intake to the adolescent with anorexia nervosa. A no-blame attitude helps limit social, emotional, physical and academic damage. The family and their child need to be prepared for the long-term management of eating disorders because of mental health comorbidity. These additional conditions need to be identified and treated.

Many children, adolescents and adults with eating disorders have anxiety, depression, evolving personality disorders and substance abuse problems. The older child with an eating disorder can progress to have problems with the stable and secure formation of personality and self. This can present later as a borderline personality disorder, a complex mental health disorder significant for its severe emotional dysregulation, impulsivity, lowered self-esteem, self-harm and associated suicide attempts.

Children and young adolescents with depression, anxiety or autism can present with the clinical markers of an eating disorder. Their underlying depression is not always recognised. It can be falsely attributed to the physical effects of extreme weight loss. Depression and starvation cause changes in cognition and motivation.

Many clinicians hold off an assessment for depression until the child is within a safe weight range. If a child tells you that they are depressed, we should listen and treat their depression, even if they have an eating disorder. The perception of the child is important.

Positive supports

Families have access to many dedicated medical, nursing and allied healthcare professionals. They are sensitive to the special needs created by eating disorders. If you are the parent of a child with an eating disorder, trust them to help your child recover. There is an excellent chance of this.

Individuals and their families share the emotional trauma of eating disorders. To better understand their impact think about post-traumatic stress disorders which are frequently talked about in the media. The aftermath of eating disorders can be a form of this disorder. It takes a lot of hard work, time, love and patience for families to recover. This is a time when families learn the value of friendship.

The experience of mental health trauma within families is not all bad. It can create positive moments, often through humour and life perspective. You get to know your child and yourself better and learn to stamp out the pettiness of life's problems.

For the parent of a child with an eating disorder, you will find comfort in the book *The Boy Who Loved Apples* by Amanda Webster. This is a story of hope, written with passion by a mother whose son had anorexia and survived. Another helpful resource for parents and adolescents is the book *Eating in the Light of the Moon – How Women Can Transform Their Relationships with Food Through Myths, Metaphors and Storytelling* by Anita Johnston, PhD.

The Butterfly Foundation is a national organisation which provides information and resources to children, adolescents, adults and families with eating disorders or early warning signs of this such as distorted body image. I have listed their website in the resource section on eating disorders.

You can't ignore eating disorders. You need to combat them early with professional help to prevent the potentially traumatic pathway of forced acute medical intervention. This can have a devastating impact on the child and their family.

Never give up on eating disorders. Your child must have great strength, resolve and determination to starve or force-feed themselves. These same qualities will help them beat the obstacles of this disorder and survive and move on to have productive and positive lives. Once your child decides to get better, they will. Always believe in your child and don't forget to love and care for yourself, your partner and other siblings.

DOs – 10 to 15 years
Do
- be available to speak with your pre-teen or teen
- talk less – to say little is to gain more
- maintain a structured family routine – provide a safety net for the anxious and autistic child
- seek professional help if your child becomes highly anxious, withdrawn or sad
- say hello to your neighbours – you will need them one day
- always love your child even if you don't like them
- show your child that you can fail too
- know that it's never too late to talk, listen and interact with your teenager
- walk away when angry, think when quiet, talk when calm

- acknowledge that it's never too late to change your parenting behaviour
- learn to forgive, forget and move on
- keep the channel of communication open and the welcome mat at the door

DON'Ts – 10 to 15 years
Don't
- try to parent alone – there is always someone to help
- practise parental narcissism
- control your child's life
- speak in anger with your child – this could make them leave home
- live your life through your child's opportunities
- forget to consult with your child about life and school choices
- place unrealistic and excessive pressure on your child to achieve academically and socially
- rescue your child – you will drown yourself
- do your child's homework
- display excessive behaviours with electronic screen time, food and exercise
- be 'Bad DADS' – bad driving, alcohol, drugs and smoking
- fail to parent
- be a reactive parent
- compete with your child – trying to dress better and swear more creatively
- make poor choices – school and home related
- fail to act
- defer parenting by keeping busy
- displace friendships with business pursuits
- forget to tell your child you are sorry

Part 8

Getting there and beyond – 15 to 25

Never give up. Never surrender.

Jason Nesmith, played by the actor Tim Allen

in the movie *Galaxy Quest*

Time to make jam and do washing

Coping with the emerging adult

The adolescent years capture the child of 13 to 15 until they reach the threshold of adulthood at 18. My mother made the best jams, marmalades and chutneys during those years. This was a useful distraction from the turmoil of this misunderstood epoch. I now understand that the unrest of adolescence can resurface during the adult years. When I see my mother stirring marmalade, I know that life is still busy.

My equivalent outlet during the adolescent years was to do lots of washing. Our house was never perfectly neat, but we always had clean and well-washed clothes. Some people find solace in gardening. You can't easily do this at midnight. The laundry, however, is the casino of the house. It has no clocks or timeframe, just a means to reflect quietly when the busyness of the day has settled.

Late adolescence and the emerging adult years is the time for parents to remain calm, compassionate and available. They have to be the parent and not slip into friendship mode. This doesn't work. Most of all, they should reconnect with their partner, peers and the interests they have neglected during the busy child–raising years.

Perception

How your adolescent tackles life will be partly determined by how they recollect their early years. Good childhood memories are the child's security blanket. Bad experiences can become their nightmares. Some children live with uncertainty. Erratic, volatile and inconsistent patterns of parenting chip away at the emotional resilience of even the strongest of these children.

Facing conflict provides opportunities to develop 'street cred' and resilience to cope with confrontation in adult life, but at an emotional cost. For the vulnerable and sensitive child, the price can be the stability of their mental health. Conflict and dysfunction are life's reality. If you are a parent who feels inadequate, scared, angry and unsupported about raising your teenage child, don't be afraid to ask for help. You are not alone.

Planning a family

I found the transition from childhood to adolescence intense. Our two girls were very close in age. Although you can't do 'designer' families, I would plan to have my children when I was around 26 to 34 years of age. Recovery time of two to three years between babies would help. Of course, I didn't do this! Having a child after the age of 36 can be exhausting. Most women have less physical energy and greater expectations as they mature.

Many couples defer their family until they perceive it to be the 'best' time for financial or career reasons. They regret their decision when they have difficulty conceiving. Fertility falls with age. It is important to factor this in when planning a family.

An older parent does not necessarily mean a better parent. Many adolescents resent having 'dinosaur' parents. The good news is that once adolescence has passed your child will nearly always acknowledge that you are the best mum or dad. Age becomes irrelevant. That moment will affirm all your hard parenting work.

Stay on the ant trail

Hang in there

Don't wish your child's adolescence away. It is important to stay calm and focus on parenting. Try to understand the language of your teenager. This means being cognisant of text speak, YouTube hits, music artists and the content of electronic games. This helps you communicate with your teenager.

My daughters have always educated me about the latest comedians and musicians, both old and new. I can recall being in the car one evening, my eyes on the road and my ears tuned to my teenage daughters' conversation about Lou Reed's song, 'Walk on the Wild Side'. I had never really 'heard' the words before. Neither had the British Broadcasting Corporation when an eon ago they let that particular song slip through their censorship net!

Driving an adolescent around introduces you to an eclectic mix of artists and music genres such as indie. My favourite reference to the genre of indie is in the Urban Dictionary. It defines indie as 'an obscure form of rock which you only learn about from someone slightly more hip than yourself'.

My daughter's definition of indie is 'that it is an independent, little heard of style of music, books or clothes that goes against the trend'. She told me that it was 'a bit like hipster', but that 'hipster was more pretentious'. Her explanation was 'that if you rode a unicycle into work, listened to vinyl and sourced organic oats from Germany, you were a hipster, but to afford the lifestyle you had to have lots of money and an Apple iPhone'.

You can learn lots about life and yourself when you're driving with your teenage child! They will force you to step outside your comfort zone. This is a good thing. There is a positive side of being the parent to the adolescent or young adult, so enjoy the experience. You are very privileged to get a chance to go on this ride. Do it, even if you don't like indie music.

Don't compete

Parents can't compete with their children. If you are the mother of a teenage daughter, keep your look current. Change your glasses, have a good haircut and upgrade your wardrobe. Teenagers get embarrassed if you turn up looking like 'try hard' vintage.

You are a person with needs. Late adolescence and the early adult years are a time when the emotional demands of your children can swamp and overwhelm you. To maintain your self-esteem, keep fit, feel good and connect with friends.

Anyone who tells you that they cruised through this period is lying. It doesn't matter how good a parent you are or how amazing your children can be. If you don't spend regular time being with family, communication will decay.

Stay cool

The language of childhood gets lost for a while during the adolescent and early adult years. It is replaced by offensive expletives and stony stares. Teenagers will swear to shock, relate to their peers and to test your reaction. For some teenagers swearing is an integral part of their learned language. When and how it is used is important.

A mother told me that her teenager in anger had typed in the words 'Fuck You' on her GPS as they were driving. There are a number of responses this could evoke. The calm or dismissive one prevents driver distraction. Humour works!

This mother made a comment to the effect of: 'Wrong destination'. She could also have said, 'I haven't downloaded that Lily Allen song yet!' I can think of plenty worse scenarios that mothers have to face. As a parent you need to pick your battles. For some parents this would be a major one. For others, it would rate a long way down their priority list.

The swearing, caustic talk of teenagers and their silent glares don't reflect the potential of the adult within. See the child; don't hear the words. If you have done the hard parenting work, you will be rewarded by your adult child engaging with you. Your teenager will return to the civility of adult conversation. During this transitional time remain the parent. Don't fall into the trap of trying to use more colourful words than your child. You will lose this contest and their respect.

Find alternative ways to vent your anger and frustration other than swearing, shouting, drinking or demeaning your child. You are their mentor and role model – not their friend. They don't have to 'like' you. Your child's future mental health depends on your ability to be the adult.

Never reject your child in anger or say the words that exile your child from their home. They may not return. It can be safer to walk away from emotional conflict when it is accompanied by physicality. You can fight for a relationship on a calmer day.

Kids at home

Dr George O'Neil, a Perth obstetrician, was a strong advocate for the use of naltrexone in the management of heroin dependency in the 1990s. He cautioned against the late adolescent leaving home to live in share 'party houses' where they would be exposed to older adults and drugs. He advised, 'Keep them at home until they are 25'.

The social milieu has changed a little. Your adult kids can't afford to leave home. A compromise is to tolerate them at home for a little longer than you hoped, educate them more about drug use, give them the emotional resilience to make good choices and be around if they don't.

Elastic parenting

Parental duty has been extended by compulsory school attendance until 17 years of age and the expectation that students enter into tertiary studies upon school completion. Kids study at home and are older before they gain financial independence. Parental retirement is deferred or exchanged for the role of caring for their own older mother or father.

Having emerging adults or even grandchildren under your roof can be difficult. Transgenerational parenting rules vary. This can create conflict between grandparents and their own children.

Parents of a dependant, adult child with a disability can feel socially isolated and even shunned by the 'normal families' around them. They are often financially disadvantaged because of loss of income through parental separation or the inability to work whilst caring for their child. This can lead to some carers becoming emotionally and physically exhausted, highly anxious or depressed.

The parent who has raised a child with a disability has a social safety net from schools; support organisations; health professionals, such as minders; extended family; and funding through government disability support schemes.

The parent of a child who develops mental distress or addiction during their teens or early adult life is often unprepared for the emotional turmoil and disruption this causes. These carers find it hard to access the appropriate medical, psychological and psychiatric support, especially if their child falls between child and adult services.

Teenage mental health

You are not alone

When a child with a mental health problem reaches 15 or 16 years of age, parents see their role as diluted. Mental health workers can step in and displace parents. They can further disrupt complex families.

A dismissive approach to parental perspective is a common complaint. Parents should seek advocacy with a professional such as a psychologist, so that they remain mentally strong. They need contemporaneous documentation of their story when family communication breaks down.

Help

Assistance is available for teenagers and the families dealing with mental distress. Depression, bipolar disorder, borderline personality disorder, anorexia nervosa, bulimia, anxiety and addiction are conditions with support and counselling services. Each state has a number of these. I have listed some helpful websites in the resource section.

Crisis presentation

For many families dealing with mental health problems, their first contact is the family doctor, child health nurse, school or the hospital emergency department.

When parents have been unable to secure help for their teenager they turn up in crisis at a large public emergency department. Their child may have overdosed on alcohol or drugs or self-harmed.

High school students from all years and particularly in Years 10, 11 and 12 are drinking alcohol regularly. Parents too often get the call to collect their 16 or 17 year old from a party to find them stoned and drunk. Sometimes kids who are semi-comatose after doing shots, mostly vodka, need to be observed medically to make sure they are breathing and their airway isn't obstructed. They are medically monitored. They could have taken substances such as ecstasy or NBOMe (N-methoxybenzyl). These drugs can cause seizures or abnormal heart rhythms.

Kids can be discharged from emergency departments without a definite management plan in place and no incentive to change their behaviour. If you find yourself sitting in an emergency department with your vulnerable child, make sure you get a proactive plan with suitable contacts and support numbers. This is an opportunity to work with your teenager to change their trajectory. Treat the crisis episode as a wake-up call.

Your child will leave the hospital department with a potential e-health record. When your teenager is well you need to discuss with them what medical information they want to withhold from being included in a future confidential electronic health record. There is concern about cybersecurity and potential access to sensitive medical and mental health data by multiple healthcare professionals and others. Your emerging adult has rights. It is their choice about what childhood and adolescent health records are included in an e-health format.

Alcohol culture

We have to work with kids to change the social culture around alcohol and drug use. This means that adults have to be more responsible about their own drinking and recreational habits. You can't prevent your teenage child from drinking alcohol if they decide they're going to drink. But you can stick to your values and rules about the use of alcohol within your home. This is an adult responsibility.

It is not legal to serve alcohol to kids under 18 years of age. It is hard to enforce this when your teenager holds an impromptu sleepover. Kids that you've never seen before conceal vodka in water bottles, or duck out of your house to retrieve hidden stashes of alcohol.

We escaped gatecrashing horror stories, but if you are not around as a parent it can easily happen.

One night our daughter held a small party. I insisted that I would be home and in the background to provide food and assistance if required. There were a couple of unfamiliar faces at the party. One girl tried to text a few friends to come over. She asked my daughter for our correct address. Our daughter joked with her and said, 'Text them that "parents at home" and "party shut down"'.

It is important that your kids learn life skills because they are going to need them. Online courses such as the Responsible Service of Alcohol and practical experience working as a waitperson, serving drinks in a bar or working at a nightclub can deter your teenager from spending money on alcohol. Keep them busy.

Parental self-worth

Don't change your shoes – your feet are still the same size
Retain your self-identity when you parent an emerging adult. Mothers care for everyone within the home and forget that they too have needs.

At a secondary school social function, I found myself next to an eloquent mother. I felt intimidated as I was a working mum and she was a stay at home mother who ran the 'perfect' household. However, as I have come to understand there is no 'perfect'. She felt inadequate as a person – socially and intellectually. She told me that her successful sons and businessman husband treated her as an attractive appendage.

I was standing there in awe of her dedication and resolve to be the best mother that her sons could possibly have. I was shocked to see that within the walls of her family home, someone had forgotten to say, 'Thanks mum', or 'I love you, mum'. These words are important for all mothers. Children and partners should never take a mother or father for granted.

Respect parents

A parent's intellect must never be denigrated as inferior should they choose parenthood as their vocation. Our society must respect and pay parents properly for undertaking, not always by choice, the responsibility and burden of child raising. This is the only unpaid 24/7 job in the world.

Parents sacrifice their time and energy to ensure that Australia reaps their investment of emotionally and socially competent people. They go out of their way to prioritise family life. Parenting is more flexible than in the past. It is not defined by set roles. Parents of all gender identities and extended family, friends, mentors and carers work together to raise healthy and happy children. This is essential if our country is to continue to flourish from the rich diversity provided by a successful multicultural society which embraces differences with tolerance.

Time for a cuppa

Adolescence requires parents to be patient and wait. Any parent who has sat for hours at a swimming or netball event would attest to this. The teenage pre-driving years describe the many hours of 'time fill' that you experience as a parent, waiting to be the chauffeur to a party or event not easily attainable by public transport.

Taking time in a busy schedule to be quiet and reflect keeps you balanced and better able to traverse this developmental stage. Parenting an adolescent is a bit like standing on the top of the advanced mogul ski run, knowing that the only way down is to face the challenge and do it, even if you have to snowplough the whole way down.

The good news is, by the time your child reaches early adulthood, you will have had lots of time to practise your parenting. If your technique is alright, you will get through this stage intact.

A friend of mine was building a new home. She became overwhelmed with the hectic demands and sought advice from a clinical psychologist. She was told when stressed to choose the slowest truck or car on the road to drive behind. If you are going to be late, use extra think time for reflection and planning. Be rested when you reach your destination.

Teenagers are invariably late. In my busy schedule this was an anxiety-provoking situation. I didn't want my kids to miss what I considered to be important appointments or events. My advice having jumped through hoops too high would be to step back more and help them face the consequences of missed events.

A medical friend was always good about defining boundaries with her kids and not changing them. If her daughter forgot her lunch or homework, she went hungry or missed getting her work marked. That was the rule. Sometimes this mother was given flak by the school. They thought her stance was too tough on a primary school student. She stuck to her decision and her child learned to take her lunch to school.

Our parenting styles initially differed. She drew her parenting boundary lines with permanent marker and I used chalk. Over time, our lines have merged and we have wonderful children with the strengths of passion, hope and aspiration. I attribute that to learned consistency, flexibility and fallibility.

You have to let go of the baton to handover

Make way for your independent child

Until our kids got their licence, life consisted of long pauses while we waited to take or collect them to and from places. A priority during this time is to get your children to drive. I thought that when this happened I would be a nervous wreck, unable to sleep or think until I heard the familiar sounds of my daughter's car returning home. The day my daughter gained her licence I had the best sleep and I haven't worried since. I felt a sense of freedom and was glad that my child had greater control over her life.

She was well prepared for driving by her dad. As part of his driving mentorship he made her change car tyres, check the tyre pressure, oil and water and fill up with petrol. She was the only student in her co-ed Year 11 class able to change a tyre.

She was prepared for independent driving. If she had an accident, it was out of our control. I just had to trust her. When she had that first accident, which all parents fear, no one was injured. The only consequence was that the car took a trip to 'Toyota heaven'. As parents we considered that a satisfactory outcome. You can buy another car, but you can't replace a child.

My kids have got their dad to thank for a number of life skills. He has always encouraged them to have a go at tasks, irrespective of gender. These included climbing up ladders from a young age to hand over tools to him while he was working on the air-conditioning units on the roof!

Our kids have also learned how to fish, snorkel, ride two-wheeled bikes, tie shoelaces and do bow lines, clove hitches and reef knots from their practical Queen Scout dad.

We have brought different strengths to the relationships we have formed with our children. We have both worked hard to instil the love of reading, writing and learning so that our children can have options and choice in their lives. We have discussed values, beliefs, tolerance and ethics. Sometimes we have failed, like all parents, but we keep trying.

I am fortunate to still hear their singing, laughter and music interrupt the silence of our home. As parents I think it is important during these emerging adult years to keep the dialogue going but not interrupt the flow of the conversation. I constantly say in my head 'less is best' when talking to my teenage girls. Trust, believe and listen to your child.

Step back

Step back and assign tasks to your children. This has a practical consequence. It allows them to grow up!

> *I still have the 'best dad'. He would always check my car when I first started driving. He would ensure that there was sufficient water and oil and that the batteries were charged. Years later, when I bought my first brand new car. I noticed white smoke pouring out from behind the car. My car had done 30,000 kilometres and was just out of warranty. I hadn't thought to have my car serviced, because my dad had always done that for me!*

Being kind to your kids and protecting them from failure can defer success. Strong parents adhere to the principle of 'tough love'. They reap the benefits of that stance. 'Tough love' can work if it is practised with fairness, consistency and balance and as long as your parenting is not controlling and rigid.

Embrace late adolescence

Try to enjoy the time you spend with an emerging adult son or daughter. Those long drives in the car provide opportunities to talk and bond with them. Just don't talk when you are in the passenger seat, your adolescent is behind the wheel and a yellow L-plate is flapping on your back window. The time to talk is when you scream 'stop' before impact with your hand within arm's distance of the handbrake.

The best road trip I took was the 250-kilometre commute with one of my daughters to her Leavers break at Dunsborough in Western Australia. I had time to speak with her and got to know her that little bit better. She asked me about my trips overseas when I was young and, grateful for the lift, listened to my choice of music for the entire journey!

Our family has always been open about life and death and the inequity and responsibility of the polarisation of wealth. Discussions have been about voluntary euthanasia, suicide, organ donation, gay marriage and abortion. The rights of the child and young adult, including intellectual property rights and the privacy of electronic health records have been debated. We have talked about self-harm, the danger of spiked drinks, alcohol shots and drugs such as ice, marijuana and NBOMe. There were lots of topics to choose from when embarking on our epic trek to Leavers. I have survived on the 'brownie points' since.

Don't be afraid of adult children

Less talk, more listening

Don't be afraid of the emerging adult within your walls. This was good advice given to me by a colleague. The other useful mantra to link to adolescence is to believe unconditionally in your child. If you don't believe 110 per cent in your child, who will?

It is important for parents to be prepared to apologise to their child when they have wronged them. Apology is necessary for healing, especially when a child has been part of an abusive relationship within their own home. It takes great courage for an adult to tell their teenager that they are sorry. When an apology is required, a parent must find that strength.

Parents need to be strong role models for their children. Kids notice how their parents cope and react. Teenagers are proud of the achievements made by their mum or dad. Family discussions which highlight the positive and negative experiences of an adult's day can also provide the teenage child with coping strategies to use in their lives.

Tenuous relationships

The relationship we form with our young child has to be re-ignited during the adolescent years. Relationships change and even in families can't be assumed to last forever. Never be complacent about family relationships. They require hard work, humility, flexibility and apology. Most of all they are bound in trust. Parents and their teenage children can grow apart during the adolescent and early adult years. We need to recognise this and think about how we can reconnect with our child.

It is a cop-out to blame technology for the social and emotional disconnection of an adolescent child. Find something in common to share with a teenage son or daughter, even if this is just a regular mealtime.

Understand the language your teenage is using to converse with on social media. Text speak is not difficult. It has been a long time since parents fell into the trap of thinking LOL was 'lots of love' and not 'laugh out loud'.

Sitting down in the same room and 'being tolerated' while your emerging adult watches a TV program or film is a start. Planned regular contact time with your teenager is better than intense one-off events. Try having a walk together or sitting down at a friendly café for a coffee and chat on a weekly basis. Your teenage child needs to see that you have made time for them. They want to hear the words, 'I love you'. Remember to say them.

Some fathers will plan a holiday with their son or daughter during the high school years. This creates a relaxed space for meaningful discussion. The holiday doesn't have to be a bribe exercised in an exotic location. It just has to be the gift of a father's time with their child. Take these opportunities, even if you are busy and distracted by your own agenda.

Keep the conversation open between yourself and your teenage child. If you are unable to do this, speak with someone who can guide you to handle your own emotions. This helps you deal better with outbursts from your adolescent.

Patient parenting

Parenting is forever. It demands work, resolve and the steadfast belief that whatever adverse circumstances your child and family face, there can be a positive outcome. Parents need to be patient and hang in there for their teenage child. As a parent you need to listen more, lecture less and communicate. Some families find that this can be done over dinner and others when driving in the car.

The habit of conversation is created early. This doesn't happen when professionals drag their young kids along with them to work at weekends. Parents are tired, stressed and busy and their child is bored. Get up earlier, work efficiently, don't stop and socialise, and get home on time. You have a child or children waiting at home for your time. That is your priority.

Families with a history of eating disorders find mealtimes stressful. Trying to have 'deep and meaningful' discussions can further cement the hate relationship a child has with food. Food refusal and the control of food intake can become even more entrenched.

You have to work out as a parent which is the best setting for communicating effectively with your child. Sometimes you are given a precious wild card opportunity to talk with a recalcitrant teenager. Grab it with both hands, listen to your child and try to shut up unless invited to speak. Never give up on your child or yourself. Always try harder, even when you've failed dismally.

Children aren't pixels, they're people

Electronic privacy

When does the electronic supervision and monitoring of children and teenagers by their parents become electronic stalking or a violation of their privacy?

I first thought about this when an 11-year-old child told me that they had lost their friend because of the use of a 'silly' nickname. This was electronically intercepted by their friend's parent. The child asked me, 'Is it right for an adult to electronically eavesdrop on a personal conversation that could have occurred in the playground?' They asked, 'Would it be right if someone opened a letter that was addressed to someone else?' I found these difficult questions to answer. Email is public communication, so what you write electronically can't be private. Even children are accountable for what they say or post.

Electronic conversations have added an extra layer of complexity to growing up. The pervasiveness and permanency of electronic messages have the potential to impact detrimentally on a person's social and emotional development. They can change the trajectory of that person's chosen life path. The misinterpretation of digital posts is particularly relevant for teenagers with high functioning autism. They frequently get the social nuances of electronic messages wrong.

The police inform us that the teenager who posts, forwards or accepts a sexualised digital image of themselves or a minor commits a cybercrime. Sending sexually provocative and nude images on social media such as Instagram are permanent digital records. These actions make teenagers vulnerable to online predators. Of greater concern, location devices on smartphones can flag a child's whereabouts.

Cybersafety

Cybersafety experts such as Susan McLean, author of *Sexts, Texts and Selfies* (2014), and Michael Carr-Gregg, a high profile psychologist, inform us about the potential traps kids face online. They instruct parents how to navigate the internet and keep children safe. This involves talking with children about online safety with the same priority as we discuss drug and alcohol use. Parents are told to keep electronic devices out of children's bedrooms and to consider the use of internet filters.

The cybersafety message is best heard and acted upon by the parents of younger children. There is a cohort of parents whose children are now over 15 years of age. They missed the opportunity to actively supervise internet usage when their children were younger. Cyber rules have to be enforced early.

It is widely reported in the media that as many as 1 in 5 Australian children from 8 to 17 years are thought to be affected by cyberbullying each year. In March 2015, in response to the increasing number of children being bullied online, government legislation was passed to assign Australia's first e-Safety Commissioner, Alastair MacGibbon. The e-Safety Commissioner has the power to demand social media sites remove offensive material, with backup under law from the courts.

Children have to know how to use technology and social media responsibly and safely. They can't do this by avoiding online communication, nor can we ethically protect them long term by using electronic tracking devices without the consent of our child.

We can actively supervise our young children's exposure to media and electronic gaming. That is our adult responsibility and a duty of care, but we need to know when to hand over this responsibility to our children.

Further information on cybersafety and cyberbullying is listed in the resource section.

The rise of the 'selfie'

The pursuit of narcissistic gratification and perfection is fuelled by the allure of the internet and the rising social status of the 'selfie'. For an increasing number of teenagers and more disturbingly for younger boys and girls, body image is disproportionately represented by online and social media sites.

Susan McLean warns us about the social dangers of inappropriate use of sites such as Snapchat, Instagram and Tinder. Genetically and environmentally vulnerable teens are prone to mental health issues due to insecurity about social and physical fit, anxiety and depression, eating disorders, self-harm and suicide.

Our newspapers print disturbing facts about teenagers as young as 13 posting sexually provocative selfies on Instagram. They highlight the trend of hypersexualised behaviours in our youth, purported to be fuelled by unsupervised and inappropriate internet access to pornography and explicit visual images depicting rough sex. This has led to the medical presentation of girls and young women with sexual injuries and anxiety.

Violence in media

Before we judge the parents of hypersexualised kids, think about how society has become desensitised to violence and sex without intimacy. High-rating TV shows such as *Game of Thrones, The Blacklist* and *Scandal* have that addictive pull. These shows have some great actors and creative value, but a high content of violence which includes torture and murder.

As adults we have the maturity and life experience to choose what we watch. Growing up, we read storybooks, sang nursery rhymes, played simple games and watched Disney movies. We are now raising, or have raised, our children and are probably ready for some mature viewing. We have to remember that our young children are not.

Sometimes teenagers become quite distressed when they are forced to watch violent or horror material in a social setting such as a sleepover. Some teenagers still prefer to watch a Disney movie. Parents have to decide what their family values are going to be in relation to the media content and exposure within their homes.

We need to think about the values that we respect within our homes and instil them in our children. When older, they can decide if, when and how they watch sexually explicit programs or play violent video games.

Some parents have no idea of the content of the electronic games played for extended hours by their children. It is not developmentally appropriate for a 10-year-old child to be playing a cruel and vicious action and adventure video game like *Grand Theft Auto*. Yet, many do.

Electronic screen exposure

Experts warn us to take a precautionary approach to screen time and content. For some kids with ADHD or autism, limited screen time can be relaxing. Too much screen time increases arousal levels and makes children aggressive.

Many of the children I see struggle to listen, hear and retain information. I wonder whether this relates to the displacement of quiet from our lives by the vast array of electronic devices we have bought into our homes. Homes now have so much 'white noise' that it can be difficult for the young child to hear a single voice.

Kids are good at processing visual information which flickers instantaneously on a bright liquid–crystal display screen, but not always good at sitting back and thinking about information and converting it into learned knowledge. This processing gap can make them appear inattentive. Social discourse had become a series of abbreviated words, linked by hash tags and shared indiscriminately with the world. There is little time for privacy and sensitivity in the way we think, write or talk about our peers.

Wayne Warburton is a psychologist who lectures about the potential for electronic addiction in kids. He talks about getting the balance of screen time right in terms of exerting the same self-control as when given a packet of chocolate Tim Tam biscuits. We can safely eat one or two, but if we consume a whole packet at once we will end up overweight. Life is about balance.

Be the boss

Electronic screen devices are integral to our lifestyle. I tell kids that they need to be the boss of them. They should have a healthy mix of play, relaxation, physical exercise, study and time left over for creative thinking.

Technology gives us great medical, scientific, educational, military, aviation and business innovations. It takes away time from reflection, being still and quiet conversation. My greatest concern is that it threatens our privacy.

We need to restore a simple lifestyle which can assimilate the pressure of technology. If life was not so busy we would feel less anxious.

How do you feel when you can't access email? What if your hard drive crashes, the computer screen turns blue and you have lost all your stored electronic data? If your heart rate increases or you feel sick by just reading this, then it is time to ponder life's priorities. Maybe it's time for an electronic curfew to be enforced in your home or office place.

In the past, banks had restricted working hours and schools closed at 3.30 pm. People respected opening hours. Sunday was a day of rest. Electronic invasion is both innovative and destructive. It has saliently eroded the social boundaries between our homes and workplaces. Homes are no longer a sanctuary. Email, smartphones, Skype and satellite phones entrap us in our work. We have forgotten the pause button between sleep and work. Life has become reactive and instantaneous. We have lost tolerance, patience and flexibility. Electronic devices should save us time but mostly they don't.

The simplicity of life eludes us. We lose time through the repetition of cut, copy and paste, rather than stop, think, reflect, write and create. These are some of the reasons why anxiety has risen in parents and is being passed onto our children.

How secure is the electronic keyhole?

Don't leave your life in 'the cloud'

Eugene Kaspersky is a cybersecurity expert and heads a global security firm. He has been quoted as saying, 'Unfortunately there is no such thing as 100 per cent security'. He allegedly said, 'If the attackers are professional enough, and have enough of a budget, I think almost every system can be hacked'.

Celebrities who entrust their private electronic data in the security of 'the cloud' and are hacked question the safety of electronic storage. The 'dark net' threatens our identity data.

Breaches occur with facsimile and paper mail, but the potential for the malicious sharing of highly personal information is greater when it can be dispersed digitally. People have already lost jobs and lucrative sponsorships because of an inappropriate text being sent by them to their boss or from an impulsive tweet which was too late to retract.

E-health

Australia's national online health record system is My Health Record, set up to provide an online medical summary accessible to healthcare professionals and hospitals. Individuals can opt out of the creation of this record or withhold specific information or access to automatically generated records from the proposed time of onset in mid-2018. Further information is provided on the Australian Government website My Health Record. The link is given under 'Other resources' in the 'Helpful reading' section of this book. Our private electronic health records form part of the electronically vulnerable storage 'cloud'. The potential for privacy breaches has already been raised. The onus is on the healthcare provider to have sufficiently robust security systems in place so that sensitive medical material is not leaked.

In 1985, when Bob Hawke was prime minister, the government tried to introduce the Australia Card, a national identification card to address tax evasion. This proved controversial and was abandoned in 1987. Yet we don't have the same level of concern about making personal and health details easily accessible electronically and conveniently to multiple government agencies.

Adolescent e-health

When e-health becomes established and functional it will be important for older children to have access to records made about them by other people. They should retain the right to opt out of these records as adolescents or young adults.

The 16-year-old girl who has independently sought medical advice about contraception or sexual health is responsible enough to have control of her own electronic health records. It is not appropriate for her parents to have access to them. We need to exercise caution as parents and healthcare professionals in what medically and psychologically sensitive material is digitally scanned into a permanent e-health record.

Medical records, particularly those created prior to the *Privacy Act*, detail family and social history. They include the names and alleged medical conditions of siblings and family members where this was felt to be medically relevant. E-health records must protect the privacy, not only of the patient who gives permission for their digital documents to be shared, but also to anyone named within them. It will be an onerous task to ensure the protection of the privacy of immediate and extended family named in retrospective, current and ongoing medical records.

Parents must be guardians of their child's medical information to protect the privacy and rights of their child. This will be a prime parental responsibility and duty of care when parents are asked to be custodians of their child's permanent digital e-health record. We need to think very carefully about the implications of not opting out of electronic health record access for our children. I hope that the law looks more closely at this area of privacy pertaining to minors.

The sharing of medical information to facilitate the best care for the patient will inevitably utilise electronic technology and will have some benefits, particularly related to the accurate documentation of pathology and radiology results and surgical details, which most patients forget. We currently have access to this information with paper records.

Teenage connectivity

Communication is more than talk

Body language is a fascinating subject. It keeps those reporting on the fabulous and famous employed. Emotional vibes, looks, glances and stares are part of social communication.

Teenage girls tell me that those same mean girls who lined the corridors of my school are still lurking. They kill confidence with a glance of disdain. A condescending look can socially exclude the vulnerable teenager from her peer group. This is social bullying and it is cruel. Social exclusion is as unacceptable today as it was when I was at high school. It should not be tolerated.

It doesn't take a university degree to read the frosty blank stare of your teenager that they are 'pissed off' with the world and with you. You just have to be brave and with great resolve and patience, wait for the thaw. It is important to be around, to have your radar up and be ready to respond when an offer to talk is made.

Teenage bullying

I recall looking after a boy diagnosed with ADHD. His mum said he was a bit quiet. It was tempting to put this down to a side effect of his medication, but listening and watching this boy I felt there was something more. It is easy for doctors, parents and teachers to miss the subtle changes that reflect emotional demise during the vulnerable teen years. I noticed the freshly healed scar on his wrist which his mother attributed to an episode of self-harm. She stated that the school were aware and had provided support and that his cutting behaviour had not recurred.

I asked this teenager what had happened. He stated that he was being bullied and felt bad about himself. He said that cutting took away those feelings and that lots of other kids were doing it, usually on concealed places such as the top of their thighs. They were also participating in the 'salt and ice challenge' and posting their results on YouTube, Tumblr and other social media sites.

The application of salt and then ice, usually on an arm, causes burning and pain. The challenge is to see how long these afflictions can be tolerated. This is a form of self-harm. It results in burns like frostbite and can cause permanent skin discolouration and damage. This teenager disclosed to his peer group what he had done. They sought adult backup by informing a teacher and asked for help. I affirmed that he had great friends.

This boy could have been from your family or mine. I have come to the conclusion, when meeting with children and their families over the years and when chatting with friends and colleagues, that there are no 'normal' families. There are just some families that are more functional than others.

Teenage lifestyles

An active, healthy lifestyle is protective for physical and emotional health. Physical activity makes us feel better because it increases our own body's 'happy chemicals' such as serotonin. Even chewing gum can increase the amount of serotonin in our saliva. If we choose a healthy lifestyle with appropriate food choices and regular exercise we will sleep and perform better. If children don't sleep well, then parents don't either. Everyone within the family gets grumpy.

Parents ask me 'How much sleep does my child or teenager need?' They require enough to keep them functioning during the day. This varies with each person. Teenagers need more sleep than younger kids. This is why it can be okay for your teenager to sleep in until 11 am on a weekend day. It doesn't mean that they are depressed or a social recluse.

The school day is totally out of sync for a teenager. Why can't we look at later starts for high school students? It doesn't make sense to drag the sleeping teenager to school. Many of them have stayed up until 1 am on Skype or messaging friends. This is the reality of teenage life today.

The best-intentioned parents struggle to win the electronic screen war with their teenager. They lost the battle when their child was very young. The widespread failure to keep smartphones, iPads and computers out of the bedroom of a teenager has nullified parental discipline.

Most of the kids I see are reliant on social media connectivity and access it unbeknown to their parents. Some households disconnect from their wi-fi after 10 pm. Parents now are better prepared to take charge of household media and computers. They collect all household electronic gadgets after 8 pm or 9 pm and charge them outside bedrooms. This needs to be an early household rule or it won't work.

I tell parents that toddlers don't need a smartphone. Some parents look aghast at me. They say, 'But they will scream and demand it, so I have to give it to them'. Parents are in charge and can take control of the electronic revolution. They should actively manage the use of electronic devices within the home so that their children and teenagers have a balanced perspective of the real and digital world.

Teenage trust

When I speak with teenagers I find that an area of great priority for them is trust. Teenagers see adults as voyeurs who control their lives and betray their trust. How many family homes manage and censor the email and phone accounts of their teenage and adult children? In the past, paper mail was delivered intact to the rightful owner. Now, email is exposed mail, too easy to intercept and interpret by others.

Most parents actively manage electronic media out of love and concern for their kids. They want to globally track their child, web cam their homes and electronically eavesdrop on the conversations and communications of their children. This is what parents are told to do. Parents have to consider the rights of their child as they transform into emerging adults and still practise their duty of care.

Concerns about breaching the trust of a child are now raised by authority figures. There are apps which give parents access to their teenage and young adult's private electronic conversations and transactions. Police have concerns that the use of these sur- veillance apps betray teenage trust.

It is better for parents to learn how to use social media and communicate effectively, honestly and openly with their child to ensure safe, responsible and proportionate electronic usage.

Parents and teachers have a responsibility to teach, mentor and instruct children about the social rules tagged to electronic media. This is the safest way for our kids to develop a pervasive social conscience that will protect them from future online bullying. It will assist them to connect safely and confidently in a digital world.

Child abuse

The ultimate betrayal of a child's trust occurs in settings of abuse. In November 2012 when Julia Gillard was Australia's prime minister, she called for a royal commission into child sex abuse. She was quoted as saying, 'Australians know…that too many children have suffered child abuse, but have also seen other adults let them down – they've not only had their trust betrayed by the abuser but other adults who could have acted to assist them and failed to do so'.

The sad reality of child abuse is that it is reported to be on the rise. Social shift is a contributor to family breakdown, child neglect and abuse. The impact of alcohol dependency and addiction on formerly cohesive and caring families is a shocking reality. The accepted social culture of alcohol hides the significance of its role in family breakdown, domestic violence and mental health problems.

Resources currently dictate the priority of care for children at risk of physical and sexual abuse. Children who suffer emotional abuse and neglect are just as vulnerable to adverse long-term emotional, social, physical and mental health problems.

School is just a small part of life

ATAR elitism

A student's Australian Tertiary Admission Rank (ATAR) doesn't define them. A 17-year-old student was quoted in an online Australian Gallup Student Poll from September 2014 as saying, 'There is a huge focus on academic studies these days, both from your school and your parents, but having said that it's important that no one sacrifices their welfare just for an ATAR'.

No one wants to read in the media about the Year 12 student who has chosen suicide and left a family bereft. Academic and personal success is not determined by a student's ATAR score, but what they are able to do with it. Some parents need to hear that.

An ATAR is earned. It belongs to the individual. If a parent feels some ownership, they have probably done too much for their child. It is not common property, so unless your child has given you permission to share their result, don't ask for their score. If they want to tell you, they will. Asking a student for their ATAR result objectifies the child.

Parental role

Principals of prestigious private schools have become increasingly outspoken on the enormous social pressures faced by today's students. In a valedictory interview, Mr Tony Little, Headmaster of Eton College in the UK, is reported to have said, 'There has been a growth in some parents vicariously living their lives through their ambitions for their children'.

As parents, we have a responsibility to mentor and guide our children. This means accepting their weaknesses, acknowledging their strengths and being there to walk alongside the path they choose, especially when this is not our choice.

Beth Blackwood, after completing eighteen years as principal of Presbyterian Ladies' College, a private girls' school in Perth, was quoted as saying, 'Too many want perfect children...allow children to fail and to learn from those failures'.

Joy Shepherd, Principal at St Hilda's Anglican School for Girls in Perth, contributed to the social commentary about education prior to her retirement. In a media interview she reflected on the decline in teacher respect and the increased parental and societal expectation on teachers. She stated that schools had been given the onerous task of adding to the curriculum: 'resilience, self-esteem, values education, healthy eating...social skills and driver education'.

Robyn Ewing, Professor of Teacher Education and the Arts at the University of Sydney, said on the online forum *The Conversation*

(12 August 2015): 'Good teachers understand that a child's social and emotional wellbeing is critical for them to learn'.

We all need to hear this and make sure that we do our job as parents and raise happy, resilient children. To do this more effectively we need to adopt a simple and uncluttered life that helps dissipate the anxiety that builds when we are busy.

ATAR perspective

An ATAR is a bonus at the completion of thirteen years of formal schooling. It facilitates access to tertiary studies as long as your child has embraced the passion to learn and self-motivate. There are many pathways for tertiary learning and vocational education options. If students through illness or misadventure bypass their ATAR, they will survive. Some will rise to be stronger in the longer term.

Encourage kids to have passion in their academic pursuit. But, they must temper this with the balance of being happy, focusing on learning and just doing the best they can. If these kids place the bar of expectation too high, they set themselves up for failure.

A Year 12 girl looked disappointed when she told me that she 'only' had an ATAR of 96.

She had failed to reach her desired score of 98. Parents can assist their child to prioritise the building of emotional and social resilience. This is the safest way of reaching an attainable goal.

Getting an ATAR of 99 is not the purpose of education, nor does it assure a student tertiary education success. School should be about gaining a sense of belonging, building the love of learning, developing a variety of skills and having a go.

There is life after school

The child who underachieves at school, for whatever reason, has to wear that consequence. This can be a significant emotional and social burden for them. Whilst we are disappointed for them, we need to maintain a healthy and responsible life perspective. The 17- or 18-year-old student has many wonderful learning years ahead. If we walk with them and help them remain emotionally strong and resilient, they will have opportunities when they are ready and prepared to have a go at future studies or pursuits.

Consider the impressive curriculum vitae of successful men and women in business, film and media, sport and other professions who were alleged not to have completed school or college. Two alleged 'college dropouts' are Steve Jobs, synonymous with Apple computers and Pixar animation fame; and Woody Allen, screenwriter, actor, director and producer.

Student engagement

Students need to keep engaged with school and learning to attain school completion. To do this, kids need to be happy and motivated and their efforts acknowledged by the teachers they like.

Why is it so hard to adopt a common sense approach to raising and educating children in a world full of resources and opportunity? What is so difficult about teaching students the fundamentals of numeracy and literacy and allowing them to play while they are still children?

When we match the learning and emotional needs of the child with their teacher, we start to see young children who want to learn. If we respected teachers more, we might encourage gifted and motivated people into the teaching profession to steer our kids along a positive learning path.

Student anxiety

Recently, politicians debated whether high school students should be forced to study maths or science as compulsory subjects in Years 11 and 12. This decision was overridden.

Forcing a senior student to do a subject, which they are likely to fail, in their last two years of school places the student at greater risk of disengaging with their academic program.

Australian high school students have high levels of exam anxiety. Journalists Natasha Bita and Laura Sullivan in an online article, 'Stressed out teens "choke" in classroom', report that 70 per cent of girls have academic performance anxiety. This can't be good for the mental wellbeing of our students.

Students would benefit from the option to choose an end-of-year exam for determining their ATAR rather than multiple stressful assessments. This would allow bright students the opportunity to learn and to extend themselves without the pressure of failures or poor marks throughout the school year. They could cram for their final exams and still have a chance to shine. 'Cramming' is what happens in real life.

Anxious students may do better with a one-off assessment, rather than the trauma of constant performance anxiety throughout their last two years of high school. School attendance would be more likely if they didn't have to fret about sitting tests every few days. They would have a chance to engage with peers and develop a sense of belonging, even if unable to face an end-of-year exam. They would at least have engaged socially at school. They can pursue tertiary studies later.

Alternative schooling

Our schools are struggling with disengaged students, many of whom have significant behavioural issues. These students can disrupt the learning environment of the classroom. They don't cope with the commitments of mainstream schooling.

In Western Australia there are a number of CARE (Curriculum and Re-engagement in Education) schools. They provide specialised support and supervision to students who remain absent from school and are at risk of falling through the education net. This is usually because of homelessness, drug and alcohol abuse, and other mental and emotional stressors. These schools aim to transition students back into mainstream schooling.

Standardised testing

Disengaged high school students miss the opportunity to learn. Students with learning disorders such as dyslexia may have low scores on Year 7 and 9 NAPLAN tests. In Western Australia, these same students struggle to pass compulsory OLNA tests and may not qualify for a high school graduation certificate.

Standardised tests discriminate against bright, anxious students, those with specific learning disorders, such as dyslexia, dyscalculia and dysgraphia, and children with ADHD and autism.

We use discriminatory testing techniques within our school system by insisting on handwritten work for examinations and written work for most assessments. In the real world we use computers. Students with a significant writing disorder, such as dysgraphia, struggle to get permission in some schools to hand in computer-generated assignments, sit tests with a scribe or answer orally.

The child who can verbally give you a correct answer demonstrates that they have understood your question, thought about it themselves and formulated a response. They have the confidence to express their ideas. This student could become a respected politician, lawyer or actor. We are not to know this. The child who hands in a high-standard essay may be a competent student but they could have had substantial parental or tutor input. How do we screen for this in our schools?

We assess intelligence on how much is written, but what is said, acted, drawn or played may be superior. Our education approach discriminates against the visual learner or the child who is exquisite at oral presentation. This is the preferred learning style of the high school student with a language impairment or ADHD. It is important that students develop good writing skills, but they should also be allowed to express themselves through a variety of media.

I challenge creative and gifted educators to think even more laterally when they teach the student with dyslexia, dysgraphia, dyscalculia, ADHD or autism. Many of these students have lifelong unrecognised language disorders. They present with problems with executive functioning and inferential high order language and reading comprehension. Psychosocial effects can occur and include anxiety, withdrawn behaviours, depression and substance abuse.

The teacher factor

John Loughran, Dean of the Faculty of Education at Monash University, shared online an analogy of the teacher's approach to students with learning needs. He said this was comparable to the doctor who has to assess their patient with medical symptoms and make a clinical diagnosis. His observation was that good teachers are able to 'find an appropriate approach for the given situation' when they are attempting to motivate and engage their student to enable learning and personal and academic achievement.

Andrew Martin, Professor of Educational Psychology at the University of New South Wales, links the importance of the good teacher–student relationship to the capacity of the student to learn, plan, self-motivate, engage and persist at their studies and participate in class. He states: 'Good teacher–student relationships are associated with lower anxiety, fear of failure and disengagement'.

There is a bank of evidence showing that teacher effectiveness is the best way to improve student performance. The impact of class size on student learning remains controversial. But, there is consensus that teaching methods appropriate for the class size need to be adopted. This reinforces the premise that to get kids to learn you have to employ teachers who can teach and want to teach, not just qualified people who have fallen into teaching by default. The same applies to parenting – it has to be from the heart and soul.

If children are already struggling at school because they have ADHD, a learning difficulty or high functioning autism they want to have a teacher who 'gets' them. These students don't cope well with the pressure of conforming to tasks with timed requirements or enforced engagement. These vulnerable students are already at risk of poor learning performance. The stress of being picked on by the teacher in front of their peers and failing by not knowing an answer is great.

Students with ADHD and learning problems often have a weakness with their processing speed. They require more 'think time'. These students should be asked a question third or fourth in line, so that they can ponder an answer. A good teacher has already worked this out.

How well a child learns and achieves at school is dependent on how the child/parent/teacher triad functions. This is more protective than class size, the aesthetics of the classroom or whether a student is allowed to raise their hand in class. A good pupil and teacher 'fit' and responsible parenting ensure the best chance for a child to complete their schooling with a successful social and academic outcome.

The student factor

South Korea is recognised for producing elite students, primed to gain entry into 'the best' universities. Their education success, however, comes at a cost. In the *Foreign Correspondent* program, 'Education Gangnam Style', aired on ABC TV in 2015, we saw exhausted students falling asleep at their desks. Students had depression and suicidal thoughts because of extreme academic pressure and 15-hour school days. Other students, who had sought an alternative education, affirmed their love of learning with teachers who saw them as individuals.

This insight into the lives of high-achieving students makes us reflect on the price of a child's education. It is not just monetary. Professor Donna Cross, former Western Australian of the Year, was quoted as saying, 'Most people don't fail in their jobs due to a lack of skills, they fail because they can't get along with others'. The difficulties some teenagers face with autism or ADHD attests to this.

In a competitive education environment, the onus is on the student to work harder, longer and smarter to reach increasingly unrealistic goals. Families and schools work best in unison to provide vulnerable students of varying abilities a balanced approach to learning.

Students will get their best results if they are self-motivated to learn, foster a passion for innovative and creative thinking, and have a sense of belonging. They need to be proud of their school and connect with their peers. Being aware of their strengths and weaknesses will assist them to develop coping strategies for the real world after school. This will allow them to become the people they aspired to be as students.

Anxiety, ADHD, SLD and autism – 15 to 25 years

Anxiety
Adolescent and adult anxiety is significant when it impacts on social and academic function. The student who survives the school years with the burden of anxiety may not successfully transition into a tertiary education course or the workforce. This is the reality of some students with autism, a generalised anxiety disorder, depression, eating disorder or evolving personality disorder.

It is never too late to get help. But, late adolescence is a time of fierce independence. The tertiary student who is struggling to complete their studies may refuse medical or psychological support.

This is a time when parents learn the long-term responsibility of raising their child. Being there for your child but stepping back and allowing them to make their own mistakes as an adult is one of the hardest lessons of parenting. You must stay resolute as a parent so that your child can be strong. This is important, as parenting is transgenerational. You hope that the child you raised will become a strong parent to your grandchild.

ADHD

Most students diagnosed with ADHD during their schooling choose to remain on stimulant medication until the completion of Year 12.

Many kids like to see how they function off medication upon school completion. The brain is a dynamic organ and so many students will be able to cope without stimulant support after finishing school or tertiary studies. For others, medication retains a useful role. Adult psychiatrists take over the care of medical management of ADHD from the paediatrician upon school completion. Adolescents with persistent symptoms of ADHD are safer when driving if they remain on medication. This has practical implications.

Tertiary institutions accommodate the additional needs of students with ADHD. They require documentation from a paediatrician or psychiatrist for any special consideration requests, such as course entry relating to attained ATAR scores.

Late adolescent and adult students with ADHD benefit from seeing a life skills coach. This is someone with expertise and experience in the management and liaison of students who have problems with executive functioning due to ADHD. They assist them with study plan techniques, organisational skills and self-esteem issues.

SLD

It is best to use words and pauses to navigate teenage and early adult life, not fists and fights. Communicating effectively and positively is difficult if you don't have the words. Australia's adult literacy levels are sub-optimal. How can we justify any child not being able to read or write after thirteen years of a formal school education?

Some government high schools provide adult literacy classes. TAFE, universities and a number of colleges offer students of all ages online and on-site bridging and catch-up courses. This provides entry avenues into diploma and bachelor courses at tertiary educational institutions. To succeed in these courses, you have to be able to read and write to a specified level of competency.

We shouldn't have to be teaching adults to read. It makes much more sense to teach our children to read.

While there is inequality in the standard of education between schools, there remains a role for selective schools. They give choice to students who want to learn and who have the ability to learn. The student's family background can preclude them attending a school that offers adequate programs in academic learning, music, drama, sport, computing and technology or visual arts.

Entry to GATE (gifted and talented education) government-funded schools opens doors for some of these students. These selective programs place students in highly competitive settings. It is vital that their emotional and social development is adequately supported. School placement is about the best fit of school for your child. Choose carefully. It is your child who has to make school their second home, not you.

Students with specific learning disorders, developmental coordination disorder, ADHD, autism, anxiety, chronic fatigue and medical illness are eligible for extra assistance. Medical documentation is provided to the school by a paediatrician or psychiatrist. Students with dysgraphia will require a report from an occupational therapist and those with dyslexia from a clinical psychologist.

Your school can apply for additional time or regular breaks for your child. You need to check with your school about the exact information required when considering an application for special consideration in assessments and exam situations. Documentation must be current. There are long waiting times to see allied health professionals. You need to be prepared, organised and current with the paperwork.

Schools and state curriculum bodies try to support all students and can be very accommodating. Tertiary institutions are extremely flexible and enthusiastic about ensuring that students engage with ongoing learning. They will consider medical and mental health burden when students apply for their courses. Some of these institutions have portfolio entry and generous mature-age entry criteria.

Autism

Many children with high functioning autism complete school and are successful in undertaking tertiary studies and challenging workplace positions. If the child with autism can cope socially with school, they will have some good strategies to face the adult world. Tertiary studies provide a further transition for them.

University and TAFE offer flexible courses to students with autism and other needs. Buddy and mentor assistance is offered. There are options for part-time, online and on-campus attendance. There are many pathways and options at all stages of learning.

Students with HFA are best to study in their home state when they first graduate from school. Familiarity and resources of home provide a safety net for the immediate period following school completion. This allows kids to be optimally supported during their late adolescence and ensures a secure base when breaking up from a serious relationship or failing their first semester exams. They are then well prepared to travel or transfer to undergraduate or postgraduate courses interstate or overseas.

Some kids relish a move away from home. This makes them grow up. Where there is family dysfunction or intractable sibling rivalry, separation of siblings can be a positive lifestyle change. If your newly graduated high school student leaves home, plan for them to have social, emotional and financial scaffolding. Better still, make sure you have raised them into a strong emerging adult by giving them emotional and social resilience. This will be their best life skill.

Children and adolescents with high functioning autism continue to struggle in late high school because of their difficulty in understanding social nuances. They misinterpret or send inappropriate text messages. Their logical, honest and blunt social discourse can be misread as rudeness or arrogance.

I have had some wonderfully challenging discussions with bright teenagers on the autism spectrum who think logically. One very blunt discourse went as follows: 'Why isn't physical and mental euthanasia legal when we can kill our unborn child?'

As we see more autism in our schools and workplaces we will need to rethink the way we communicate with each other. With the intrusion of social media and smartphones, the social gap between neurotypicals or so-called 'normal' people and those with autism is closing. We need to be less judgemental and more understanding of young adults with autism and accommodate their social discrepancies in our schools and workplaces.

The important things in life

A sense of belonging

How we cope with adult life and relationship has a lot to do with how we perceive our role and purpose. We require a strong sense of self, a knowledge of what we represent and an understanding of how we fit in.

This became apparent to me when I attended a school reunion. One of the past students who turned up had been expelled in the early high school years. She just wanted to see how the school had got on without her! Although a successful and mature adult she sought to reconnect with her formative roots. She wanted to show us that there is life after school.

Part-time work for teenage students is a great way to instil self-discipline, motivation, leadership skills, team building and values. We bemoan the commercialism and monopoly of big service retailers. But, they have an important role in the socialisation of our youth. For some teenagers, the self-esteem, purpose, remuneration and social experience from working facilitates their path through adolescence into adulthood.

The opportunity to serve burgers, roast chicken and fresh food may be the first time they have had to follow rules and instructions. There is great benefit in working six or eight hours each week during the latter school years. Too much work can be counterproductive and affect study and peer socialisation. It also springboards kids into the adult workplace, so that when they turn 18 and are studying, they already have a curriculum vitae that says, 'I am employable'.

Social disconnect

Social media has altered the way we communicate. How we connect with people and the art of face-to-face conversation remains important. Teenagers who have left school and enrolled in tertiary courses can feel lonely and disconnected. Many tertiary students are not part of a consistent cohort of students during their undergraduate studies. This reflects a trend of choosing online study above physical attendance on campus.

Some courses insist that mandatory time is spent on campus. Others don't require any on-site time. Online study has a pivotal role in engaging some students, assisting mature age and isolated students, as well as those with physical or mental health needs, but it doesn't promote social cohesiveness.

In what can be considered a paradox, Google, which allows us to explore and learn in isolation, comes up with many of its innovations by encouraging its staff to work through personal interaction. Their Googleplex model provides communal working and leisure areas to facilitate a sense of belonging. This fosters creative thinking and innovation.

There is increasing momentum for humans to connect more to their peers, to reflect on the beauty of nature and the art of self-awareness and personal meditation.

A sense of belonging is more powerful than our passions or beliefs. It is thought to be protective of our mental and physical health and even our longevity. As parents, educators, sport and extracurricular club and community members, our task is to give kids a sense of belonging. If we work together to do this, then our teenagers are less likely to seek acceptance in cults, radicalised groups and gangs, or engage in self-harm and drugs.

Kindness

Our grown-up children take with them the values we give them. Sometimes these get lost for a while, but our roots and family ties remain strong. By being patient we will recognise kindness, honesty, respect, courtesy and compassion in the children we have raised. Of all these values I consider kindness the most valuable. Whether your child is in a relationship, at work, studying or with family, they need this basic human emotion.

If kids can't be kind to themselves, they will have difficulty caring and understanding the feelings of others.

As parents we hope that our children choose a kind partner. We want their teachers and mentors to be compassionate and thoughtful, especially if our children have mental health issues, learning disorders, autism, physical illness or disabilities. When they enter the workplace we hope that peers and bosses also respect this value.

The gender gap

Women can't always have it all

Inequality of women in the workplace is reflected by the much discussed 'gender pay gap'. This is created by the allocation of predominantly male boardroom and senior administration positions and male-dominated surgical operating theatres. Film and screen gender bias exists and women are denigrated in the jobs they are forced to seek. Inequality occurs when the balance of power within the workplace is tipped.

Women have to keep fighting for equal monetary and value recognition. This doesn't mean that women can't stand firm with their male colleagues. But, they often have to strive harder and longer to reach a position of prestige and power. Women have to fight for their jobs and justify their positions.

Women continue to fight for position and acknowledgement in their chosen profession. I have listened to women such as Ita Buttrose talk about her challenges within media and publishing, and Julia Gillard recount angry confrontations with male peers. The Academy Award–winning actor Anjelica Huston in her book, *Watch Me – A Memoir,* provides the insight that even fame can't protect the vulnerability of being female in a harshly competitive world. It is still not a level playing field for women in the workplace.

Australia has produced some powerful women in politics, law, education, medicine, business and religion. Julia Gillard, Nicola Roxon, Penny Wong, Tanya Plibersek, Kate Ellis, Julie Bishop, Peta Credlin and Sarah Hanson-Young form an imposing bank of political women. They have worked ruthlessly hard. I often think of their families, and the pressures each of them must have faced at some stage.

Juggling work and children

It is very difficult to juggle motherhood or mentorship and a professional life which involves constant public scrutiny. This can be done, but there always has to be a compromise. Professional work can displace full-time motherhood. Considerable planning and support are required to ensure that children receive sufficient care, nurture and time.

Proxy carers such as early childcare workers, nannies, grand-parents or friends can fulfil the child's immediate needs. But, the child who is sick, lonely, anxious or depressed may just need some time with their mum or dad. It is heartbreaking for a parent not to be available to provide nurture in times of crisis.

A paediatric friend of mine said that you get the best hugs from your child when they are sick. I recall the time my daughter had ear, nose and throat surgery as being a special time. I got to spend some close time, reading to her, listening to her stories and sharing hugs. These intimate moments can be lost when parents get too busy in their working lives.

When you commit to parenthood you can't predict the specific needs of your child. You could have an easygoing child who goes with the flow and has a relatively uncomplicated childhood course. Sometimes a child becomes acutely or chronically ill with a physical or mental health problem. They may be diagnosed with autism, an intellectual disability or learning disorder. This changes the priorities and working structures within families.

When I have spoken with senior medical colleagues on the cusp of retirement, the comment I hear most is 'I wish that I had spent more time with my family and friends'. These sentiments, expressed by caring paediatricians, are worthy of contemplation.

I have done the hard yards and missed those magic childhood moments, the dress-up day at kindy, the first swimming lesson, the parent day at school or school assembly. It is a harsh reality of being a professional mother. I haven't been able to have it all.

When you embark on a career path that has rigid training and working requirements it is important to pause and consider whether you really want to step through this particular door. If you do, think and plan about how you can best juggle the dual roles of parenthood and a demanding career.

Some women are nearly able to 'have it all'. I admire them for their great resilience and determination. They are indebted to the people who work with them backstage, so that they can go on with the show. Raising children needs a lot of help and the recognition that the task becomes exponentially tougher as children grow from childhood into adolescence.

Anne-Marie Slaughter

Anne-Marie Slaughter was the first woman director of policy planning at the US State Department. She also had a 14-year-old son. She was faced with the dilemma of maternal conflict over 'work–family balance'. When she made the choice to leave her job she challenged other women to consider that with society's current economic and social structure, women 'can't have it all'. This viewpoint was reported in *The Atlantic* in 2012 in the article, 'Why Women Still Can't Have It All'.

She proposed that until women have sufficient power through equal representation on corporate boards and in executive positions, they won't have the power to change society so that women can have it all.

If you are the parent of a teenage girl, consider the possibility that within her lifetime she will live in a society with the choice to work in an equal workplace with men. More importantly, your daughter will have the choice to be fulfilled as a mother should she not wish to seek corporate glory.

At present, Anne-Marie Slaughter's observations are that this is only possible if you are 'superhuman, rich or self-employed'.

Covert childhood oppression

There will always be bigger footsteps to follow
The ongoing royal commission into institutional responses to allegations of child sex abuse, announced by Julia Gillard in 2012, has shocked Australians. It has provided a platform of support to those affected and affirms their emotional strength and resilience despite the grip of adversity.

Respected public figures, themselves the victims of child sexual abuse, have stood up to tell the new generations of child abuse victims that they do not carry the burden of blame and shame and should not feel fault. It is important that a sincere and meaningful apology is given for the healing of the victimised children of developmental trauma. This allows them to rebuild their self-esteem and their lives. Sadly, this is not possible for some children.

In Western Australia, Eoin Cameron, well loved as a former ABC radio icon and federal parliamentarian, gave us a sombre and poignant moment on-air. He divulged that he was a victim of institutionalised sex abuse. His courageous decision to share his story of deep emotional trauma gave many men the strength to come forward and declare that some adults had failed in their duty of care to protect the sanctity of childhood.

When we reflect on man's journey in a future world, the sins against innocent children will be firmly ingrained on the tombstone of humanity.

Any parent must feel the pain emanating from the stories we are now hearing about the abuse of trust from hallowed religious, educational, media and other respected institutions. It is also important to recognise the positive efforts by caring mentors who have worked with children within those same walls. It is crucial that they fulfil their vocation with impeccable integrity if trust is to be restored.

The mantle of mentorship

To travel hopefully is a better thing than to arrive.

Robert Louis Stevenson

You never parent alone

When we work with children and families we talk about the village effect – the need for everyone to be involved with nurturing and caring for children. Integral to the success of the village model is the mentor who can be a life shaker, maker or breaker.

The person who makes the greatest difference to a child's life is the ordinary parent, teacher, neighbour or grandparent. A simple act of kindness, compassion and belief in a young person can change a life.

My mother taught me to read. She has always been my greatest educator and moral conscience. The mentorship message I have for my children is to tell them that their toughest battle as women will be the right for freedom of speech and lifestyle. I want them to have resilience and soul. They will need conviction of spirit, knowledge and power of an education and support of their peers so that they can live in a world where they have choice and are respected.

I was fortunate to have great teachers whose giftedness and innovation made me think laterally and allowed me to believe that as a young girl I could do something with my life.

As a young doctor I received guidance, training and support from many caring and competent physicians and surgeons.

Every parent accepts a mantle of support when they face the responsibility of caring for their child. You will never be alone.

Mentors

Strong men and women who work in the arts mentor kids. Film, theatre, music and the visual arts provide a positive focus for our young adults. Teenagers aspire to be the next Jennifer Lawrence, Cara Delevingne, Zac Efron, Leonardo DiCaprio, Emma Watson, Margot Robbie, Matt Damon, Justin Bieber, Kristen Stewart, Liam Hemsworth, Robert Pattinson, Selena Gomez, Logan Lerman or Emma Stone.

Dreams, passion and time spent as a teenager groupie provide purpose, goal and motivation. Kids need an interest separate from school. It connects them with like-minded peers. This is part of teenage socialisation.

Parents have little real contact with their teenagers. Online social connectivity, peers and idols have the greater impact during this transitional period. The media is influential in determining social trends. They foster tolerance within groups of people, including our youth.

Sitcoms and rom-coms such as *Modern Family* and *The Big Bang Theory* normalise and respect differences. The film *Still Alice*, based on Lisa Genova's book, confronts dementia. The Netflix series *13 Reasons Why*, based on Jay Asher's bestselling novel, is a passionate, brave and controversial portrayal of the challenging topics of rape culture, cyberbullying and suicide that we must discuss with teenagers today.

Films such as *The Imitation Game* make a political and social statement about the barbaric treatment and atrocious social judgement of male homosexuality. Film has a voice. It is called social justice. Visual media makes a difference as to how young people treat their peers.

Famous and successful people are a part of a child and young adult's life. But, it is the mentorship of the quiet achiever that remains most influential. Educators fulfil a pivotal role in the upbringing of children. If you listen to adults speak, invariably they acknowledge the teacher who made a difference.

DOs – 15 to 25 years
Do

- live by the philosophy that life means living in the present moment
- remember – life isn't a movie watched in the rear-vision mirror; it's the story that is about to happen
- learn patience, tolerance and humility when you have children
- accept your faults and be prepared to change your behaviour
- continue to be consistent, calm and reflective in your parenting
- work together with your child or children, even when you are in separate households or blended families
- keep in contact with family and accept their help when it is offered
- be the adult, not the friend
- try to listen more and say less
- take up an invitation from a teenage son or daughter – have a coffee or go to a movie
- avoid rigid controls when parenting teenagers
- be prepared to say sorry to your child, to your partner and to yourself

DON'Ts – 15 to 25 years
Don't

- give up on your teenager
- ever be afraid of your child
- judge someone by their appearance and overlook their potential
- engage in reactive, kneejerk parenting
- be a rigid and controlling parent
- adopt complacent parenting

- electronically stalk your teenager
- talk money and finances in front of your children
- respond impulsively to your angry child – wait for them to calm down and then have a conversation
- drive bad (angry), sad, tired, distracted or with drugs and alcohol on board
- compete with your child; you will always be older, uglier and not as smart

Part 9

Waving bye-bye

I held her close and she was mine,
A stranger now, it would take time.
She held my hand. She knew my name.
I saw a smile and when I called; she came.

I took her to school, tucked her in at night.
We shared some tales, some laughs and fights.
But, one day I woke, and she was gone.
An empty giggle in a house, alone.

Then she called my name.
I listened and heard.
She shared her thoughts, and fear-filled words.
We sat quite close, in this sudden calm.
And, I glimpsed the woman she had become.

A poem by a mother and her child

Parenting is for the long haul

Hard yakka

Parenting is hard work. There are times when you will go around singing the lyrics: 'Sometimes you're the windshield, sometimes you're the bug', from Mark Knopfler's song, 'The Bug'. You will get through those days.

I've written about children and the way that small steps can take them far, as long as they have someone to guide them. If parents do their job, children will cope and take large leaps into life as emotionally resilient adults. They will be able to manage life's hardships.

I am not an expert in parenthood, but I do have expertise and knowledge in the way children grow and learn. My words are for parental reflection and consideration. Parents can choose what commentary is helpful and discard that which is not.

I have been entrusted with the life experiences of children and their families. This responsibility is to be treasured, respected and honoured. I have had the gift, honour and privilege of caring for my children and the children of others. I will keep trying to do my best and to do better.

Whilst my stories mirror the path trekked by some parents they are not intended to divulge the specific sensitivities of any one child, parent or family. This includes my husband and adult children whose privacy I respect. Where I have named a mentor, colleague or friend, I have done so with the intent to thank them for their guidance and role in my life and indirectly in the lives that I share.

I hope that these heartfelt tales and clinical observations will provide some comfort and relief for those parents who carry the burden of guilt, regret and disempowerment. I have walked in your shoes.

We can't live life backwards. Who knows what life would have been lived through a different sliding door? Life needs to be lived looking forward through the front window and not glancing back over the road already driven. Some days our lives are in shambles but there will be those days when we grasp our dreams.

Paulo Coelho, a Brazilian lyricist and novelist, wrote, 'It isn't what you did in the past that will affect the present. It's what you do in the present that will redeem the past and thereby change the future'. Whatever this life holds for ourselves and for our children, it should be a life worth living.

One of the 'perfect' mothers I met during my daughters' primary school years told me once that family faults stay at home. Families fight to protect their integrity. This is their strength and weakness. We must help families grow strong roots and through failure be better at raising resilient children, adolescents and adults.

The best of luck with your parenting. Have fun, love your children and enjoy the ride. You may as well. It's too late to get off!

Epilogue

Catch you on the flip side.

Ron Howard's film *Apollo 13*

Orson Welles was an American actor, remembered for his presence and the words he left behind. He is alleged to have said, 'If you want a happy ending, that depends, of course, on where you stop your story'.

I am going to stop my story right here. It's here and now, and not there and then.

Part 10

Helpful reading

There are books and resources which can assist with parenting. Even the discovery of one helpful parenting tip is worth the browse.

Resources

People

Seek support from extended family, friends, neighbours, teachers, the GP, paediatrician, child psychiatrist, clinical and school psychologist and allied health providers. Speech pathologists provide literacy support – not just help with the way kids talk.

Parenting

Websites

www.aap.org – The American Academy of Paediatrics (AAP) is a parent and clinician resource for a number of childhood and adolescent neurodevelopmental and behavioural problems. Topics include media and electronic use, anxiety and ADHD.

www.childrenandmedia.org.au – The Australian Council on Children and the Media (ACCM) 'promotes healthy choices and stronger voices in children's media'.

www.generationnext.com.au – Generation Next is an authoritative body that advocates for children and teenagers. It targets teachers, allied health professionals and parents. It tackles bullying, anxiety, depression, eating disorders and electronic screen addiction.

www.health.gov.au – The Commonwealth Department of Health and Ageing provides tips for parents and useful helpline contacts for each of the states and territories. They produce booklets on parenting advice for Kids 1–4 years, Kids 5–11 years, Adolescents and Parents.

www.ngala.com.au – Ngala provides early parenting and early childhood services and supports. This website includes information on Ngala DadsWA. It encourages fathers to be active in parenting their kids.

www.parentline.com.au – Parentline is a secure phone advisory and counselling service for families in Queensland and the Northern Territory.

www.raisingchildren.net.au – The Raising Children Network is an Australian parenting resource for children from birth to 15 years. Good tips on ADHD, autism and anxiety.

www.tresillian.org.au – Tresillian provides early parenting support to families in New South Wales and Victoria. A good resource for parents to deal with common problems during infancy and the early years, as well as support for postnatal depression.

www.tweddle.org.au – The Tweddle Child and Family Health Service provides access to intervention services with health professionals and vulnerable families who face challenges during pregnancy and the early school years.

Books
Brooks, R. & Goldstein, S. 2001, *Raising Resilient Children,* McGraw-Hill, New York.

Carr-Gregg, M. 2014, *Strictly Parenting – Everything You Need to Know about Raising School-Aged Kids,* Penguin Group, Australia.

Dent, M. 2016, *Real kids in an unreal world: How to build resilience and self-esteem in today's children…*, Pennington Publications, Murwillumbah, NSW.

Fowler, C. & Gornall, P. 1996, *How to Stay Sane in Your Baby's First Year – The Tresillian Guide,* Revised edn, Simon & Schuster, NSW, Australia.

Fuller, A. 2013, *Tricky Kids,* HarperCollins, Australia.

Lashlie, C. 2008, *He'll Be OK – Helping Adolescent Boys Become Good Men,* HarperCollins, London.

Murkoff, H. & Mazel, S. 2015, *What to Expect in the First Year,* 3rd edn, HarperCollins, Australia Pty Ltd.

Murkoff, H. & Mazel, S. 2013, *What to Expect in the Second Year,* HarperCollins, Australia.

Sax, L. 2015, *The Collapse of Parenting: How We Hurt Our Kids When We Treat Them Like Grown-Ups,* The Perseus Books Group, New York, United States.

Infections in pregnancy

Websites
www2.health.vic.gov.au/hospitals–and–health–services/
patient–care/perinatal–reproductive/neonatal–ehandbook/
infections – Chicken pox (varicella zoster), cytomegalovirus, Group B Streptococcus, Herpes simplex virus (HSV), listeria, parvovirus, rubella, syphilis and toxoplasmosis.

www.uptodate.com/contents/genital–herpes–simplex–virus–
infection–and–pregnancy?topicK. – Genital Herpes simplex virus (HSV) and pregnancy.

www.virologyresearch.unsw.edu.au/programs/cmv/ –
Cytomegalovirus infection.

en.wikipedia.org/wiki/Ignaz_Semmelweis – This website credits the physician Ignaz Semmelweis as being the first doctor to make the connection between the practice of hand washing and fewer infections in women following delivery.

Physical challenges

Websites

www.abilitycentre.com.au – The Ability Centre, previously known as the Cerebral Palsy Association.

www.movegrowengage.com.au – The Western Australia website for Developmental Coordination Disorder. This condition affects a child's movement, balance, posture and coordination.

Learning and disability

Websites

www.arrowsmithschool.org – The Arrowsmith Program is an intensive cognitive program that uses neuroscience research to change the learning pattern of students with specific learning disabilities such as dyslexia. It is implemented in a number of schools in Canada and around the world.

www.betterstart.net.au – Better Start for Children with Disability program outlines government funding for approved medical conditions.

www.cogmed.com.au and www.junglememory.com – Working memory programs that aim to retrain brains to think and process better.

www.dragonnaturallyspeaking.com.au – *Dragon Naturally Speaking* is a voice-recognition software. It is a helpful tool for students with dysgraphia. It helps them convert oral expression into the written form.

explicitinstruction.org/ – The website for the text and DVD series by Anita L. Archer and Charles A. Hughes. This book provides a systematic and direct approach for effective teaching across a range of student age groups.

www.loveandreilly.com.au – Love and Reilly, together with Pelican Talk and Multimedia Speech Pathology, have produced an iPad app called *Speech Sounds for Kids!* This assists children to learn about phonemic awareness, consonant sounds, the use of gestures, social cues and more.

www.nessy.com – *Nessy* is an electronic interactive literacy aid which comes with apps and a choice of UK and world and US and Canada versions. It is aimed at students from 5 to 16 years with dyslexia.

www.parentbooks.ca – Website detailing a number of helpful texts for educators and parents. *Calm, Alert, and Learning: Classroom Strategies for Self-Regulation* is a book by Stuart Shanker, a leading Canadian expert on self-regulation.

www.speedtypingonline.com and www.rapidtyping.en.softonic.com – Downloadable touch-typing tutor software programs. These are worthwhile for students with hypermobility and dysgraphia.

www.3plearning.com/uk/spellodrome and www.mathletics.com.au – Spellodrome and Mathletics are two learning instruments used widely in Australian primary schools from kindergarten to Year 12.

www.wordshark.co.uk – WordShark is a computer program to assist children with reading and spelling problems. It can be adapted for home and school use.

www.wordwizard.com – WordWizard is a spelling and vocabulary program which employs Australian voices.

Books

Andrade, J. (ed.) 2001, *Working Memory in Perspective,* Psychology Press Ltd, UK.

Engelmann, S. 1999, *Teach Your Child to Read in 100 Easy Lessons,* Simon & Schuster, New York.

Halsted, J. W. 2009, *Some of My Best Friends Are Books – Guiding Gifted Readers from Preschool to High School,* Great Potential Press, US.

Hatte, J. 2012, *Visible Learning for Teachers – Maximizing Impact on Learning,* Routledge, New York.

Levin, D. E. & Carlsson-Paige, N. 2006, *The War Play Dilemma,* 2nd edn, Teachers College Press, New York.

Mackay, N. 2011, *Taking the Hell Out of Homework,* SEN Marketing, UK.

Packiam Alloway, T. 2011, *Improving Working Memory – Supporting Students' Learning,* SAGE Publications, London.

Rimm, S. 2008, *Why Bright Kids Get Poor Grades and What You Can Do About It,* 3rd edn, Great Potential Press Inc, US.

Robinson, K. & Aronica, L. 2015, *Creative Schools*, Penguin Books, New York, USA.

Rowe, A. 1997, *Oz Mnemonics – Memory Aids for Spelling Irregularly Spelt Words for Teachers and Parents,* Focus Educational Resources, South Australia.

Ruff, D. 2005, *5 Levels of Gifted,* Great Potential Press Inc, US.

Silverman, L. 2002, *Upside-Down Brilliance – The Visual-Spatial Learner,* DeLeon Publishing, Denver, Colorado.

Walker, T. 2017, *Teach Like Finland*, W. W. Norton & Company, Inc., New York, USA.

Speech and language

Websites
https://dsf.net.au/ – The Dyslexia-SPELD Foundation Literacy and Clinical Services site for children and adults with language and learning difficulties.

www.speech-language-therapy.com – The professional and evidence-based website of Dr Caroline Bowen, author of *Children's Speech Sound Disorders*. It is an excellent resource for parents and speech therapists for a number of childhood speech presentations such as stuttering.

Music

Websites
www.bridgestomusic.com.au – Early childhood music classes in Sydney, New South Wales.

www.cottagemusicjunior.com – Early childhood music classes in Perth, Western Australia.

www.musicworksmagic.com – Early childhood music classes in Melbourne, Victoria.

www.music.uwa.edu.au/community/jms – Music for children from 18 months to 12 years.

www.pianoeasy.com.au – A different way of learning music, without the traditional adherence to note reading.

Anxiety and depression

Websites
https://13reasonswhy.info/ – a global online go-to mental health crisis site for viewers of the Netflix series 13RY who experience self-harm or suicidal thoughts.

www.aap.org – The AAP's website provides excellent information for clinicians and parents on childhood anxiety and its management.

www.anxiety.org – Anxiety.org is a helpful US website with articles about childhood anxiety, including separation anxiety and phobias. Articles are written by specialists from diverse backgrounds.

www.beyondblue.org.au – Beyondblue is a national organisation which has raised the awareness and decreased the stigma of mental health problems due to anxiety and depression in the age group 12 to 25 years.

www.bpdaustralia.com/family-connections-1/ – The National Education Alliance Borderline Personality Disorder (NEA–BPD) Australia coordinates the research-based Family Connections program for those in a relationship with someone diagnosed with a borderline personality disorder.

www.brave-online.com – An online, interactive self-help program for children, teenagers and adults who suffer with anxiety.

www.headspace.org.au – Headspace is a National Youth Mental Health Foundation established by government to address mental and physical health problems, work and study issues and drug and alcohol dependency. It targets young people aged 12 to 25 years.

http://helpingminds.org.au – HelpingMinds is a free counselling service in Perth, Western Australia. It offers support to adults and young people from 8 to 18 years with a family member affected by mental illness. Previously known as Arafmi (WA), the Association of Relatives and Friends of the Mentally Ill.

www.lifeline.org.au/ – Lifeline crisis support and suicide prevention site. They provide 24/7 phone access to people in distress. The lifeline number is 13 11 14.

http://au.reachout.com/ – ReachOut is an excellent online support site about mental distress.

www.sane.org – SANE Australia, the National Mental Health Charity, which assists people struggling with mental health issues.

www.smilingmind.com.au – The Smiling Minds app introduces young people to the concept of mindfulness and quiet thinking.

http://suicideprevention.com.au/get-help/ – The Suicide Prevention website lists 24/7 resources (current 2017). They include Lifeline 13 11 14, Hold On To Life @ the Australian Suicide Foundation, 1800 HOLDON (1800 465 366) and Suicide Callback 1300 659 467.

https://suicidepreventionlifeline.org – United States residents 24/7 crisis line for mental distress. Has Spanish and deaf and hard of hearing access.

www.youthbeyondblue.com, www.youthfocus.com.au and the Black Dog Institute, www.blackdoginstitute.org.au, and Lifeline Australia at www.lifeline.org.au – Other state and national services that provide crisis advice and counselling.

Books

Adelson, J. L. & Wilson, H. E. 2009, *Letting Go of Perfect – Overcoming Perfectionism in Kids,* Prufrock Press Inc, Texas, US.

Burns, E. 2009, *Nobody's Perfect – A Story for Children About Perfectionism,* Magination Press, Washington DC.

Chansky, T. 2008, *Freeing Your Child from Negative Thinking,* Da Capo Press, US.

Crist, J. 2004, *What to Do When You're Scared and Worried: A Guide for Kids,* Free Spirit Publishing Inc, US.

Daniels, S. & Piechowski, M. 2009, *Living with Intensity,* Great Potential Press Inc, US.

Fonseca, C. 2011, *Emotional Intensity in Gifted Students – Helping Kids Cope with Explosive Feelings,* Prufrock Press Inc, US.

Huebner, D. 2006, *What to Do When You Worry Too Much – A Kid's Guide to Overcoming Anxiety,* Magination Press, Washington, DC.

Mackay, H. 2013, *The Good Life – What Makes a Life Worth Living?* Pan Macmillan Pty Ltd, Australia.

Rapee, R., Wignall, A., Spence, S., Cobham, V. & Lyneham, H. 2008, *Helping Your Anxious Child,* Raincoast Books, Canada.

Semple, D. J. & Lee, J. 2011, *Mindfulness-Based Cognitive Therapy for Anxious Children: A Manual for Treating Childhood Anxiety,* New Harbinger Publications, California.

ADHD

Websites

www.apa.org/topics/adhd/ – The American Psychological Association (APA) covers practical and research areas on ADHD in children and adults.

www.additudemag.com – The magazine ADDitude's website provides information on ADHD for families.

www.cdc.gov/ncbddd/adhd/ – The Centers for Disease Control and Prevention (CDC) includes recommendations made by the AAP for the paediatric management of ADHD. Parents, teachers and carers can download ADHD checklists from a number of online sites such as this one.

www.chadd.org – The nationally recognised authority Children and Adults with ADHD (CHADD) supports and informs parents and those who care for kids with this condition.

www.cogmed.com and www.junglememory.com – Cogmed and Jungle Memory are electronic programs devised to improve working memory.

http://ww2.health.wa.gov.au/Articles/S_T/Stimulant-medicines –
The Government of Western Australia Department of Health
website with information on the prescribing of stimulant
medication, including dexamfetamine, lisdexamfetamine and
methylphenidate.

http://ladswa.nationbuilder.com/ – LADS is the Learning and
Attentional Disorders Society of WA. It provides information
and advocacy support for those affected by ADHD and
associated conditions.

www.nhmrc.gov.au/guidelines-publications/mh26 – The
National Health and Medical Research Council (NMHRC) has
downloadable (PDF) information on ADHD.

www.nimh.nih.gov/health/topics/attention-deficit-hyperactivity-
disorder-adhd/index.shtml – The National Institute of Mental
Health (NIMH) is a good ADHD resource.

www.uptodate.com/patients – The Up-To-Date public website
gives advice about ADHD to families, including information on
stimulant medication.

Journals
Green, E. 2017, 'The comorbidities that exacerbate ADHD',
Journal of the Australian Medical Association WA (Medicus), February,
pp. 30–1.

Books
Barkley, R. 1998, *Attention Deficit Hyperactivity Disorder – A
Handbook for Diagnosis and Treatment,* 2nd edn, The Guilford
Press, New York.

Guare, R., Dawson, P. & Guare, C. 2012, *Smart but Scattered Teens: The 'Executive Skills' Program for Helping Teens Reach Their Potential,* The Guilford Press, US.

Kutscher, M. L. 2014, *Kids in the Syndrome Mix of ADHD, LD, Autism Spectrum, Tourette's, Anxiety and More!,* 2nd edn, Jessica Kingsley Publishers, London.

Schwarz, A. 2016, *ADHD Nation – The Disorder. The Drugs. The Inside Story,* Little, Brown, Great Britain.

Silva, Prof D. & Toner, M. 2017, *ADHD Go-to Guide – Facts and Strategies for Parents and Teachers,* UWA Publishing, Western Australia.

Autism

Websites

www.AutismApps.org.au – The Autism Association of Western Australia has introduced a site to navigate the most appropriate educational and fun apps for children with autism.

http://www.autism-help.org – A helpful resource for families with a child with autism.

www.autism.org.au – Provides an autism advisory service, early intervention, workshops and other services. Each state has relevant online resources for children diagnosed with ASD.

www.carolgraysocialstories.com – New website of Carol Gray's Social Stories.

www.dss.gov.au – The government's Department of Social Services which has superseded the role of FaHCSIA (Families, Housing, Community Services and Indigenous Affairs).

www.fragilex.org – Provides information on the genetic condition of fragile X.

www.growingtogether.com.au – The website for the Helping Children with Autism (HCWA) package provided by the Department of Social Services (DSS).

www.humanservices.gov.au – Provides details about the eligibility of funding of services for children with autism, such as the Carer Allowance.

www.pdasociety.org.uk – Website of the Pathological Demand Avoidance Syndrome awareness society.

www.raisingchildren.net.au/children_with_autism/children_ with_autism_spectrum_disorder.html – The Raising Children Network parenting site.

www.sst-institute.net – Website for the Secret Agent Society, a social skills program for children with HFA from 8 to 12 years.

www.tonyattwood.com.au – The website of Tony Atwood, a psychologist with expertise in the area of high functioning autism and Asperger syndrome.

Books
Attwood, T., Grandin, T., Faherty, C., Wagner, S., Iland, L., Wrobel, M., Bolick, T., McIlwee Myers, J. & Snyder, R. 2006, *Asperger's and Girls,* Future horizons Inc, Canada.

Baker, J. E. & Smith Myles, B. 2003, *Social Skills Training – For Children and Adolescents with Asperger Syndrome and Social-Communication Problems,* Autism Asperger Publishing Company, Kansas, US.

Baron-Cohen, S. 2008, *Autism and Asperger Syndrome – The Facts,* Oxford University Press, UK.

Holliday Willey, L. (ed.) 2003, *Asperger Syndrome in Adolescence,* Jessica Kingsley Publishers, London.

LeGoff, D., De La Cuesta, G., Krauss, G. & Baron-Cohen, S. 2014, *Lego Based Therapy: How to Build Social Competence Through Lego-Based Clubs for Children with Autism and Related Conditions,* Jessica Kingsley Publishers, London.

Lord, C. 2006, *Rules,* Scholastic Press, US.

Notbohm, E. 2005, *Ten Things Every Child with Autism Wishes You Knew,* Future Horizons Inc, US.

Notbohm, E. 2006, *Ten Things Your Student with Autism Wishes You Knew,* Future Horizons Inc, US.

O'Reilly, B. & Smith, S. 2008, *Australian Autism Handbook,* Jane Curry Publishing, NSW.

Silberman, S. 2015, *NeuroTribes: The Legacy of Autism and the Future of Neurodiversity,* Allen & Unwin, Australia.

Willey, L. (ed.) 2003, *Asperger Syndrome in Adolescence,* Jessica Kingsley, London.

Rare diseases support groups

Websites
www.arcan.org.au – Website of ARCAN – Australian Rare Chromosome Awareness Network.

http://gardn.org.au/ – The WA-based website for GaRDN – Genetic and Rare Disease Network.

www.rarechromo.org – The website for Unique, a UK-based group for understanding chromosome disorders.

www.rarevoices.org.au – Provides online resources for Rare Voices Australia.

Eating disorders

Websites

www.thebutterflyfoundation.org.au – The Butterfly Foundation is a national organisation which provides information and resources to children, adolescents, adults and families with eating disorders or early warning signs of this, such as distorted body image.

www.eatingdisordersinfo.org.au – This website is an innovative resource which targets vulnerable young adults.

www.maudsleyparents.org/ – A site for the parents of eating disordered children.

www.tred.org.au – The website for TRED (Tasmania Recovery from Eating Disorders). This resource provides recovery group support for adolescents and adults of 18 years and above and family support for carers of those of any age with an eating disorder.

Books

Johnston, A. 2000, *Eating in the Light of the Moon – How Women Can Transform their Relationships with Food through Myths, Metaphors and Storytelling,* Gurze books, Carlsbad.

Treasure, J., Smith, G. & Crane, A. 2007, *Skills-Based Learning for Caring for a Loved One with an Eating Disorder – The New Maudsley Method,* Routledge, East Sussex.

Webster, A. 2012, *The Boy Who Loved Apples,* The Text Publishing Company, Melbourne.

Bullying and cyberbullying

Websites

www.amf.org.au – The Alannah and Madeline Foundation funds initiatives to protect children from violence and bullying. Innovations include eSmart Digital Licences for all year 6 Australian students to help combat cyberbullying.

www.bullyingnoway.gov.au – Bullying. No Way! is a schools-based initiative set up by the Safe and Supportive School Communities (SSSC) working group.

www.cybersafetysolutions.com.au – Website of Susan McLean, cybersafety expert and author of the book *Sexts, Texts & Selfies.*

www.esafety.gov.au – A resource for internet and mobile phone safety advice.

www.itstimewetalked.com.au – A parent cybersafety resource.

www.ncab.org.au – The National Centre Against Bullying (NCAB) combines expertise from law, education and business to tackle bullying from school to the workplace.

Other resources

Websites

www.250k.org.au – Allergy website, funded by government. A valuable resource for those 250,000 people between 12 and 25 years with life threatening allergy. It also shows how to give an EpiPen injection when someone is having an anaphylactic reaction to a food or other allergen.

www.adf.org.au – The Alcohol and Drug Foundation website.

www.aedc.gov.au – Website of the Australian Early Development Census (AEDC).

http://www.aihw.gov.au – The Australian Institute of Health and Welfare provides statistics in a number of healthcare areas, including child health, development and wellbeing.

www.childrenandmedia.org.au – Rating and review online site which advocates for safe media exposure for children.

www.commonsensemedia.org – Provides age-appropriate reviews of electronic media.

www.digitalnutrition.com.au – Psychologist Jocelyn Brewer's online resource to promote healthy digital choices for children, adolescents, students, parents and educators.

www.disability.wa.gov.au – Information about the National Disability Insurance Scheme (NDIS) – WA.

www.downsyndrome.org.au – Online resource for families who care for a child with Down syndrome.

www.ehealth.gov.au – Electronic health record information.

www.fds.org.au – Family Drug Support Australia provides assistance to families affected by drug and alcohol use.

www.gamesforchange.org – A program which uses digital games to facilitate responsible social change for individuals or community groups.

www.health.gov.au – The Department of Health's website with full indexing to cover services, treatment plans, access plans and mental healthcare. Accesses to the 2015 report, *The Mental Health of Children and Adolescents – Report on the Second Australian Child and Adolescent Survey of Mental Health and Wellbeing.*

www.health.vic.gov.au/neonatalhandbook/conditions/jaundice-in-neonates.htm – Neonatal eHandbook website which lists information on common neonatal conditions from A to Z. Includes facts about jaundice in the first two weeks of life under 'J'.

www.humanrights.gov.au/our-work/childrens-rights – This resource gives access to a child-friendly version of the Children's Rights Report 2014 and useful submissions, including those in the report on intentional self-harm and suicidal behaviour in children.

www.humanrights.gov.au/submissions-intentional-self-harm-and-suicidal-behaviour-children – This link accesses 140 written submissions made in 2014 to Megan Mitchell, the National Children's Commissioner's report on intentional self-harm and suicidal behaviour in children. (Submission 66 made by the author, Dr Elizabeth Green).

www.immunise.health.gov.au/internet/immunise/publishing.nsf/Content/pregnant-women – The Immunise Australia Program website details vaccination access to women during their pregnancy.

www.itsonus.org – A site to increase awareness around sexual assault.

www.kidsafe.com.au/crguidelines – Website for Kidsafe Child Restraint Guidelines.

https://www.moneysmart.gov.au/life-events-and-you/families/teaching-kids-about-money – An excellent government website which teaches children how to manage money and their finances for now and their future.

http://www.mychildwithoutlimits.org/plan/dental-care/ – Speech Therapy Resources / My Child Without Limits site. Provides information about caring for teeth in babies and young children.

https://myhealthrecord.gov.au/internet/mhr/publishing.nsf/content/home – The Australian Government's website about My Health Record, an online medical summary which with patient permission can be accessed by a range of healthcare professionals.

www.natureplaywa.org.au – A way to connect kids with nature and encourage them to take risks and learn resilience.

http://nbpsa.org – The website for the Neurodevelopmental and Behavioural Paediatric Society of Australasia. It provides online information for patients and practitioners.

www.ranzcog.edu.au/college-statements-guidelines.html – The Royal Australian and New Zealand College of Obstetricians and Gynaecologists – College Statements and Guidelines.

www.rednose.com.au/section/safe-sleeping – Advice about SIDS prevention.

http://stillaware.org – Advice about stillbirth prevention.

www.thyroid.org – The American Thyroid Association's website gives good public information about iodine deficiency.

www.tsh.org.au – Telethon Speech and Hearing website in Western Australia.

http://www.uptodate.com/contents/clinical-manifestations-and-diagnosis-of-coarctation-of-the-aorta – Online medical resource for best practice information. This site is accessed by paid subscription and login. However, parent resources are readily accessible on the UpToDate website.

www.psychologyconcepts.com/still-face-experiment/ – A free psychology resource which illustrates the still face experiment; well known for its demonstration of maternal-infant bonding.

http://www.movegrowengage.com.au/dcd-resources – Western Australian, government supported initiative to share information with parents, teachers and clinicians about developmental coordination disorder. Symptomatic children have motor problems which affect their ability to write, balance and dress. This condition impacts independence, emotional confidence, social participation and learning.

Bibliography

Alongside reading

Aesop's Fables, 1994, Wordsworth Editions Limited, Herdsfordshire.

Alborough, J. 1994, *Hide and Seek,* Candlewick, United States.

Alborough, J. 1998, *There's Something at the Letterbox,* Walker Books, London.

Allen, P. 1994, *Clippity-Clop,* Penguin Books, Australia.

Allen, P. 2009, *Is Your Grandmother a Goanna?* Penguin Group, Australia.

Allen, P. 1982, *Who Sank the Boat?* Penguin Books, Australia.

Argent, K. & Weld, A. 2001, *Dinnertime!* Working Title Press, South Australia.

Bang, M. 1999, *When Sophie Gets Angry – Really, Really Angry…,* The Blue Sky Press, New York.

Bemelmans, L. 1997, *Madeline's Rescue,* Scholastic Children's Books, London, UK.

Berenstain, S. & Berenstain, J. 1997, *Inside Outside Upside Down,* Random House Inc, New York.

Bita, N. 2007, *Fuzzy-Wuzzy Wombat and other Rhymes,* Koala Book Company, Mascot.

Bradman, T. & Chamberlain, M. 1989, *Look Out, He's Behind You,* Methuen Books, Great Britain.

Carle, E. 1999, *The Very Clumsy Click Beetle,* Philomel Books, New York.

Carle, E. 1970, *The Very Hungry Caterpillar,* Hamish Hamilton Ltd, Great Britain.

Carlisle, R. & Launchbury, J. 1995, *The Letterland ABC,* Collins Educational, London.

Dodd, L. 1995, *Slinky Malinki, Open the Door,* Penguin Books Ltd, England.

Fox, M. 2015, *Baby Bedtime,* Penguin Aus, Australia.

Fox, M. 1998, *Koala Lou,* Penguin Books, Australia.

Fox, M. 1989, *Shoes from Grandpa,* Scholastic Australia Pty Limited, Gosford.

Fox, M. 1998, *Tough Boris,* Penguin Books, Australia.

Fox, M. 2014, *Where is the Green Sheep?* Penguin Aus, Australia.

Fox, M. & Rawson, O. 2010, *A Giraffe in the Bath,* Penguin Aus, Australia.

Gibbs, M. 2007, *The Complete Adventures of Snugglepot and Cuddlepie – including Little Ragged Blossom and Little Obelia,* HarperCollins Publishers (Australia) Pty Ltd.

Hill, E. 2015, *Spot Bakes a Cake,* Penguin Books Ltd, United Kingdom.

Machin, S. & Vivas, J. 1997, *I Went Walking,* Omnibus Books, South Australia.

Majid, E. 2011, *A Sausage Went for a Walk*, Fremantle Press, Western Australia.

McBratney, S. 1994, *Guess How Much I Love You?* Walker Books Ltd, London.

Milne, A. A. 1927, *Now We Are Six,* Methuen & Co Ltd, London.

Milne, A. A. 1924, *When We Were Very Young,* Methuen & Co Ltd, London.

Moroney, T. 2006, *When I'm Feeling Kind,* The Five Mile Press Pty Ltd, Victoria.

Ramage, J. & Hickman, E. 2008, *Tuart Dwellers,* WA Naturally Publications, Australia.

Ramage, J. & Peterson, L. 2004, *Eyes in the Night,* UWA Press, Western Australia.

Ramage, J. & Wilson, M. 2012, *Deepsea Whale Rescue,* Department of Environment and Conservation, Government of Western Australia.

Ramage, J. & Wilson, M. 2010, *Stranded,* Black Dog Books, Australia.

Rosen, M. & Oxenbury, H. 1997, *We're Going on a Bear Hunt,* Walker Books Ltd, London.

Seuss, D. 2012, *Dr. Seuss's ABC,* HarperCollins Publishers Ltd, London.

Seuss, D. 2011, *Fox in Socks,* HarperCollins Publishers Ltd, London.

Seuss, D. 2012, *Horton Hears a Who!* HarperCollins Publishers Ltd, London.

Seuss, D. 2010, *Green Eggs and Ham,* HarperCollins Publishers Ltd, London.

Seuss, D. 2010, *How the Grinch Stole Christmas!* HarperCollins Publishers Ltd, London.

Seuss, D. 2011, *Oh, The Places You'll Go!* HarperCollins Publishers Ltd, London.

Seuss, D. 2011, *One Fish Two Fish Red Fish Blue Fish,* HarperCollins Publishers Ltd, London.

Seuss, D. 2010, *The Cat in the Hat,* HarperCollins Publishers Ltd, London.

Seuss, D. 2011, *The Cat in the Hat Comes Back,* HarperCollins Publishers Ltd, London.

Seuss, D. 2012, *The Lorax,* HarperCollins Publishers Ltd, London.

Seuss, D. 2012, *There's A Wocket in my Pocket,* HarperCollins Publishers Ltd, London.

The Nursery Rhymes of Winnie the Pooh, 2000, Penguin Books, Australia.

The Three Billy Goats Gruff, 1993, Ladybird Books Ltd, UK.

Waddell, M. 1990, *Can't You Sleep Little Bear?* Walker Books, London.

Whelan, S. 2015, *Don't think About Purple Elephants,* Exisle Publishing, Australia.

Wild, M. 1997, *Our Granny,* Omnibus Books, South Australia.

References

American Psychiatric Association. 2013, *Diagnostic and Statistical Manual of Mental Disorders*, 5th edn.

Andre, C. 2014, *Mindfulness*, Rider, Great Britain.

Arcelus J., Mitchell A. J., Wales J. & Nielsen S. 2011, 'Mortality rates in patients with anorexia nervosa and other eating disorders. A meta-analysis of 36 studies', *The Journal of the American Medical Association*, vol. 68, no. 7, pp. 724–31.

Asher, J. 2007, *13 Reasons Why*, Razorbill, Penguin Group Inc., USA.

Bagshaw, E. 2015, 'We don't have time for mental health: teachers', *The Sydney Morning Herald*, 4 May.

Banks, A. 'Retiring judge rues meth-caused misery', *The Weekend West*, 24–25 April 2015

Barrett, R. 2015, 'Thousands of Australian students lack hope for future with only a third optimistic about landing good job, Gallup poll shows', *ABC News* [online], 1 March. Available: <http://www.abc.net.au/news/2015-03-01/students-lack-hope-for-future-says-poll-gallup-australia/6269960> [Accessed 22 August 2015].

Barrowclough, A. 2015, 'Why are so many young rugby league players taking their own lives?', *The Weekend Australian Magazine*, 30–31 May.

Bent, C. A., Dissanayake, C. & Barbaro, J. 2015, 'Mapping the diagnosis of autism spectrum disorders in children aged under 7 years in Australia, 2010–2012', *The Medical Journal of Australia*, vol. 202, no. 6, pp. 317–20.

Bita, N. 2015, 'Calling "time out" on generation stress', *The Weekend Australian*, 13–14 December, p. 21.

Bita, N. 2015, 'Click bait; kids at risk as sexualized behaviour becomes "new normal"', *The Weekend Australian,* 30–31 May 2015.

Bita, N. 2015, 'Curriculum shifts focus to core skills', *The Weekend Australian –Inquirer,* 8–9 August, p. 4.

Bita, N, 2015, 'Students won't be forced to do maths', *The Weekend Australian –* Nation, 30–31 May, p.6.

Bita, N. 2015, 'Teaching kids the language of the future', *The Weekend Australian,* 7–8 November, p. 22.

Bita, N. & Sullivan, L. 2017, 'Stresses out teens 'choke' in classroom, *The West Australian* [online], 20 April. Available: <https://thewest.com.au/news/wa/stressed-out-teens-choke-in-classroom-ng-b88450618z> [Accessed 16 May 2017].

Blunt, L. 2012, *Beating the Bullies,* Jane Curry Publishing, Australia.

Bowlby, J. 1988, *A Secure Base,* Routledge, New York.

Branley, A. & Hermant, N. 2015, 'Child neglect cases across Australia increase; services failing to support at-risk children', *ABC News* [online], 6 June. Available: <http://www.abc.net.au/news/2015-06-06/child-neglect-on-the-rise-across-Australia/6526260> [Accessed 22 August 2015].

Brown, A., Shifrin, D. L. & Hill, D. L. 2015, 'Beyond "turn it off": How to advise families on media use', *AAP News* [online], October. Available: <http://aapnews.aappublications.org/content/36/10/54.full.pdf+html> [Accessed 17 October 2015].

Burridge, K. 2010, *Gift of the Gob – Morsels of English Language History,* HarperCollins Publishers, Australia.

Carney, M. 2015, 'South Korean education success has its costs in unhappiness and suicide rates', *ABC news* [online], 16 July.

Available: <http://www.abc.net.au/am/content/2015/
s4255647.htm> [Accessed 31 August 2015].

Carr-Gregg, M. 2007, *Real Wired Child,* Penguin Aus,
Australia.

Carr-Gregg, M. 2014, *Strictly Parenting*, Penguin Group,
Australia.

Carr-Gregg, M. 2013, *The Princess Bitchface Syndrome: Surviving
Adolescent Girls*, Bolinda, Australia.

Castellanos, F. X. 2015, 'Is adult-onset ADHD a distinct
entity?', *American Journal of Psychiatry* [online], 1 October.
Available: <http://ajp.psychiatryonline.org/doi/abs/10.1176/
appi.ajp.2015.15070988?journalCode=ajp> [Accessed
29 November 2015].

Child and Youth Health, 'Bedwetting', *Raising Children Network*
[online], Available: <http://raisingchildren.net.au/articles/
bedwetting_(cyh).html> [Accessed 23 August 2015].

Conversation, The 2014, 'Expert panel: what makes a good
teacher', *The Conversation* [online] 12 August. Available:
http://theconversation.com/expert-panel-what-makes-a-
good-teacher-25696 [Accessed 22 August 2015].

Cooke, Kaz. 2007, *Girl Stuff − Your Full-On Guide to the Teen
Years,* Penguin Group, Australia.

Cooper, W. O. et al. 2011, 'ADHD drugs and serious
cardiovascular events in children and young adults',
The New England Journal of Medicine', 17 November,
pp. 1896–903.

Crawford Adams, J. 1976, *Outline of Orthopaedics,* 8th edn,
Churchill Livingstone, Great Britain.

Dent, M. 2003, *Saving Our Children from Our Chaotic World,*
Pennington Publications, Australia.

Denton, A. *Enough Rope* (Video recording), 24 September 2007, ABC Video.

Department of Health 2015, 'Education and Prevention', *The mental health of children and adolescents* [online], August, Australian Government. Available:<http://www.health.gov. au/internet/main/publishing.nsf/Content/mental-pubs-m-child2> [Accessed 1 January 2016].

Doran, M. 2015, 'Use of cage for boy with autism at Canberra school prompts call for national education standard', *ABC News* [online], 3 April. Available: <http://www.abc.net.au/ news/2015-04-03/experts-slam-need-to-cage-boy-wth-autism-at-canberra-school/6369470> [Accessed 23 January 2016].

Duff, F. J., Reen, G., Plunkett, K. & Nation, K. 2015, 'Do infant vocabulary skills predict school-age language and literacy outcomes?' *Journal of Child Psychology and Psychiatry,* vol. 56, no. 8, pp. 848–56.

Duffy, C. & Mendes, J. 2015, 'Police caution parents against using new Teensafe app to spy on children's smartphone activity', ABC news [online], 14 April. Available: <http:// www.abc.net.au/news/2015-04-13/police-caution-against-new-teensafe-spying-app-for-parents/6389660> [Accessed 30 August 2015].

Dunn, A. 2017. *The New Puberty*, Melbourne University Press, Melbourne, Australia.

Engelmann, S. 1999, *Teach Your Child to Read in 100 Easy Lessons*, Simon & Schuster, New York.

Ewing, R. 2015, 'Drexel Releases National Indicators Report on Autism & Adolescent Transitions', *Drexal Now* [online], 21 April. Available: <http://drexel.edu/now/archive/2015/ April/Autism-Indicators-Young-Adult-Transition/> [Accessed 30 August 2015].

Fatemi, S. H. 2011. 'Fragile X mental retardation protein levels are decreased in major psychiatric disorders' [online], 1 December. Available: <http://www.ncbi.nlm.nih.gov/pmc/articles/PMC2981618/> [Accessed 28 August 2015].

Fraiberg, S. H. 1959, *The Magic Years: Understanding and Handling the Problems of Early Childhood,* Charles Scribner's Sons, New York.

Gallego, G., Goodall, S. & Eastman, C. 2010, 'Iodine deficiency in Australia: is iodine supplementation for pregnant and lactating women warranted?' *Medical Journal of Australia,* vol. 192, no. 8, pp. 461–3.

Gates, M. 2017, 'I spent my career in technology. I wasn't prepared for its effect on my kids', The Washington Post [online], 24 August. Available:< https://www.washingtonpost.com/news/parenting/wp/2017/08/24/melinda-gates-i-spent-my-career-in-technology-i-wasnt-prepared-for-its-effect-on-my-kids/?utm_term=.6e122f700eb4#comments> [Accessed 29 August 2017].

Gervay, S. 2000, *I am Jack,* HarperCollins, Australia.

Gladwell, M. 2008, *Outliers: The Story of Success,* Little, Brown and Company, US.

Goleman, D. 2005, *Emotional Intelligence – Why It Can Matter More than IQ,* 10th Anniversary edn, Bantam Books, New York.

Greenfield, S. 2008, *ID – The Quest for Meaning in the 21st Century,* Sceptre, Great Britain.

Griffin, C. 2015, 'Probiotics in obstetrics and gynaecology', *ANZJOG,* vol. 55, no. 3, pp. 201–9.

Hagerman, R. & Hendren, R. 2014, *Treatment of Neurodevelopmental Disorders – Targeting Neurobiological Mechanisms,* Oxford University Press, USA.

Hiatt, B. 2014, 'Challenge to lure cream to teaching', *The West Australian* [online], 3 October. Available: <https://au.news.yahoo.com/thewest/wa/a/25176862/challenge-to-lure-cream-to-teaching/> [Accessed 5 October 2015].

Hiatt, B. 2015, 'Too many want perfect children: principal', *The Weekend West*, 3–4 October, p. 3.

Hilliard, M. 1958, *A Woman Doctor Looks at Love and Life,* Macmillan & Co Ltd, Australia.

Hjelmgaard, K. 2014, 'Internet of Threats: Q&A with Eugene Kaspersky', *USA Today* [online], 6 November. Available: <http://usa.kaspersky.com/about-us/press-center/in-the-news/internet-threats-qa-eugene-kaspersky-usa-today> [Accessed 22 August 2015].

Hurst, H. 2015, 'Pushy parents endanger children's mental health', *The Times* (London, England), May 18, p. 13.

Huston, A. 2014, *Watch Me,* Simon & Schuster UK Ltd, London.

Illingworth, R. 1979, *The Normal Child – Some Problems of the Early Years and Their Treatment,* 7th edn, Churchill Livingstone, New York.

Jaspers, T. et al. 2009, 'Pervasive refusal syndrome as part of the refusal-withdrawal-regression spectrum: critical review of the literature illustrated by a case report', *Eur Child Adolesc Psychiatry* [online], 21 May. Available: <http://www.ncbi.nlm.nih.gov/pmc/articles/PMC2762526/> [Accessed 30 August 2015].

Jeffers, S. 2007, *Feel the Fear...and Do It Anyway,* 20th edn, Ballantine Books, New York.

Jensen, B. 2010, *Investing in Our Teachers, Investing in Our Economy,* [online], Gratton Institute, Melbourne. Available: <http://grattan.edu.au/wp-content/uploads/2014/04/057_report_education_investing_teachers.pdf> [Accessed 30 August 2015].

Johnston, B. 2012, 'Meet WA's Australian of the Year', *Offspring* [online], Autumn. Available: <http://issuu.com/sallytravis/docs/os_autumn_to_issuu> [Accessed 30 August 2015].

King, M. 2017. *Being 14*, Hachette Australia, Sydney NSW.

Kutscher, M. 2014, *Kids in the Syndrome Mix of ADHD, LD, Autism Spectrum, Tourette's, Anxiety and More,* 2nd edn, Jessica Kingsley Publishers, London.

Lake, J. K., Perry, A. & Lunsky, Y. 2014, 'Mental Health Services for Individuals with High Functioning Autism Spectrum Disorder', *Autism Research and Treatment* [online], September. Available: <http://www.hindawi.com/journals/aurt/2014/502420/> [Accessed 17 October 2015].

Lask, B. 2004, 'Pervasive refusal syndrome', *BJPsych Advances,* vol. 10, no. 2, pp. 153–9.

Laurie, V. 2015, 'Worlds worst: fetal alcohol hits one in eight', *The Australian* (National Australia), 17 January, p. 1.

Legge, K. 2015, 'Making the switch', *The Weekend Australian,* 18–19 July, pp. 12–16.

Levin, D. E. 2013, *Beyond Remote-Controlled Childhood, Teaching Young Children in the Media Age,* National Association for the Education of Young Children, US.

Mansell, W. 2010, 'Poor children a year behind in language skills' [online], Available: <http:www.theguardian.com/education/2010/feb/15/poor-children-behind-sutton-trust> [Accessed 31 August 2015].

McLean, S. 2014, *Sexts, Texts & Selfies,* Penguin Group, Australia.

Moroney, T. 2006, *When I'm Feeling Kind,* The Five Mile Press Pty Ltd, Victoria.

Morton, R. 2016, 'Autism doctor shopping warning', *The Australian,* 19 January, p. 1.

Neven, R. S. 1996, *Emotional Milestones,* ACER Press, Melbourne.

O'Leary, C. 2015, 'Probiotic plan for baby safety', *The West Australian,* 14 October 2015, p. 3.

Packiam Alloway, T. 2011, *Improving Working Memory – Supporting Students' Learning,* SAGE Publications Ltd, London.

Parnell, S. 2015, 'NDIS experts to help half of all kids with autism disorders', *The Australian* – Nation, July 29, p. 7.

Parry, T. 2005, 'Assessment of developmental learning and behaviour problems in children and young people', *Medical Journal of Australia,* vol. 183, no. 1, pp. 43–8.

Peters, S. 2013, *The Chimp Paradox,* Jeremy P. Penguin Group, US.

Petersen, C. 1950, *The Adventures of Pipkin the Elf,* Ward Lock & Co Ltd, London & Melbourne.

Philosophy & Philosophers. 2012, *Woody Allen Quotes* [online], Available: <http://www.the-philosophy.com/woody-allen-quotes> [Accessed 5 October 2015].

Pinker, S. 2015, *The Village Effect – Why Face-to-Face Contact Matters,* Atlantic Books, London.

Pownall, A. 2015, 'Sleep problems keep kids awake', *The Weekend West,* 25–26 April.

Pownall, A. & Millimaci, G. 2015, 'Money raised helps to ease pain of patients', *The Weekend West,* 17–18 October, pp. 8–9.

Prescott, S. 2015, *Origins – Early-Life Solutions to the Modern Health Crisis,* UWA Publishing, Crawley, Western Australia.

Raine-Fenning, N. 2014, 'Hard evidence: does fertility really "drop off a cliff" at 35?' *The Conversation* [online], 15 July. Available: <http://theconversation.com/hard-evidence-does-fertility-really-drop-off-a-cliff-at-35-29113> [Accessed 30 August 2015].

Riley, C. & Williams, S. 2015, *Growing Great Kids,* HarperCollins, Australia.

Robinson, K. 2009, *The Element – How Finding Your Passion Changes Everything,* Penguin Group, US.

Rodgers, S. 2015, 'Generation stressed being left behind', *The Australian* – Nation, June 20, p. 5.

Roedell, W. 1984, 'Vulnerabilities of highly gifted children' *Roeper Review,* vol. 6, no. 3, pp. 127–30.

Rollins, A. 2015, 'Forcing GPs to adopt half-baked e-health record a dud idea: AMA', *Australian Medicine,* September, pp. 14–15.

Schmidt Neven, R. 1996, *Emotional Milestones,* ACER Press, Melbourne.

Science Daily. 2012, 'Brain development delayed in ADHD, study shows' [online], 30 July. Available: <http://www.sciencedaily.com/releases/2012/07/120730094822.htm> [Accessed 30 August 2015].

Scott, S. 2015, 'Number of children seeking help for mental health problems doubles since 1998, landmark survey shows', *ABC News* [online], 7 August. Available: <http://www.abc.net.au/news/2015-08-07/landmark-youth-mental-health-survey/6679320> [Accessed 25 October 2015].

Shaw, P., Lerch, J., Greenstein, D., Sharp, W., Clasen, L., Evans, A., Giedd, J., Castellanos, F. X. & Rapoport, J. 2006, 'Longitudinal mapping of cortical thickness and clinical outcome in children and adolescents with attention-deficit/hyperactivity disorder', *Arch Gen Psychiatry,* May, vol. 63, no. 5, pp. 540–9.

Sheridan, M. D. 1998, *From Birth to Five Years,* ACER Press, Melbourne.

Sheridan, M. D. 1999, *Play in Early Childhood,* 2nd edn, ACER Press, Melbourne.

Silva, D., Colvin, L., Glauert, R., Stanley, F., Srinivasjois. R. & Bower, C. 2015, 'Literacy and numeracy underachievement in boys and girls with ADHD', *Journal of Attention* [online], August. Available: <http://jad.sagepub.com> [Accessed 19 August 2015].

Simmons, A. 2015, 'Pushy parents stress out children, Eton head says', *BBC News* [online], 18 May. Available: <http://www.bbc.com/news/education-32779506> [Accessed 22 August 2015].

Simple English Wikipedia, 'Woody Allen' [online], Available: <https://en.wikipedia.org/wiki/Woody_Allen> [Accessed 5 October 2015].

Simsion, G. 2013, *The Rosie Project,* Text Publishing, Australia.

Slaughter, A. M. 2015, *Unfinished Business,* Penguin Group, Australia.

Slaughter, A. M. 2012, 'Why Women Still Can't Have It All', *The Atlantic,* July/August, pp. 1–21.

Swan, D. 2015, "Hackers exploiting the 'internet of threats'", *The Australian* – IT, June 9, p. 27.

Thorpe, I. 2012, *This Is Me,* Simon &Schuster Pty Ltd, Australia.

Tillett, A. 2015, 'Child allergies linked to mum's diet', *The West Australian*, 9 November, p. 7.

Twenge, J. M. 2017, iGen – Why Today's Super-Connected Kids Are Growing Up Less Rebellious, More Tolerant, Less Happy – and Completely Unprepared for Adulthood – and What That Means for the Rest of Us, Simon and Schuster, New York, NY 10020.

US National library of Medicine. 2014, 'Pregnancy and Substance Abuse', *Medline Plus* [online], 10 August. Available: <https://www.nlm.nih.gov/medlineplus/pregnancyandsubstanceabuse.html> [Accessed 30 August 2015].

Warburton, W. & Braunstein, D. (eds) 2012, *Growing Up Fast and Furious,* The Federation Press, Sydney.

Whitehouse, A. 2016, 'NDIS provides basis for streamlining autism diagnoses', *The Australian*, 19 January, p. 10.

Whitehouse, A. & Alvares, G. 2015, 'New "wonder drug" not a panacea for autism' *The West Australian,* 29 October, p. 20.

Whiting, N. 2015, 'Mental health: survey finds high rates of stress in children', *AM with Michael Brissenden* [online], 5 October. Available: <http://www.abc.net.au/am/content/2015/s4324968.htm> [Accessed 6 October 2015].

Widmer, R. & Wright, G. 2005, *Paediatric dentistry*, 5th edn, Kids Health Department, The Children's Hospital, Westmead.

Yeoman, W. 2015, 'Open minds', *Weekend West Magazine,* 14–15 February.

Part 11

Appendix

Infections that can make your baby sick

Screening for infection in early pregnancy

During the first thirteen weeks of pregnancy, an initial blood test is taken to check for hepatitis B, human immunodeficiency virus (HIV) and syphilis. Sex, blood contact or a blood transfusion can transmit these infections. Screening is done for rubella, a mild childhood disease. In pregnancy it causes devastating effects for the unborn child.

TORCH infections

Syphilis and rubella are part of the TORCH group of in-utero infections associated with neonatal mortality (death) and neonatal and later childhood morbidity (chronic illness and disability).

These serious congenital infections can affect the baby before they are born. TORCH is an acronym that stands for toxoplasmosis, other (syphilis), rubella, cytomegalovirus (CMV) and herpes simplex virus (HSV). Some people would include HIV infection and varicella zoster (chicken pox).

TORCH infections can affect important body organs such as the brain, eyes, ears, skin, liver, spleen and blood. They can result in seizures (fits), brain damage, intellectual and learning disabilities, loss of hearing and vision, rashes, liver and spleen damage, and abnormal bleeding.

Syphilis and HSV are sexually transmitted infections (STIs), referred to in the past as sexually transmitted diseases (STDs). They can be prevented by 'safe sex' practices. Condoms are cheap, simple to use and protective. But, if you are trying to get pregnant you won't be using them! You could be unknowingly at risk of these diseases. This is where trust, communication, respect, honesty and education of yourself and your partner is important.

Education regarding the nature of STIs remains an important preventive public health issue for women of childbearing age. If you have one STI, you could have others, which include HIV, hepatitis B, hepatitis C and chlamydia infection.

Numerous infections can affect the unborn baby. They include enteroviruses. These are virulent viruses which can cause meningitis, severe gut infections and sepsis in the newborn baby. Other 'nasties' include varicella zoster virus (chicken pox), parvovirus B19 (slapped cheek) and listeria, a rare bacterial infection. We don't routinely screen for these infections, but be aware of them if planning a pregnancy.

Listeria

Listeria is the term used to refer to the bacteria *Listeria monocytogenes*. It is found in some foods. In humans it can cause the rare but harmful disease listeriosis. If transmitted to your unborn child during pregnancy it can cause miscarriage, premature labour or the sudden death of your baby, known as stillbirth.

Foods which may contain listeria include paté, meat pastes, processed meats such as ham and salami, chicken, cold smoked seafood such as salmon, oysters and sushi, pre-cooked prawns, pre-prepared salads and soft-serve ice-cream. Soft cheeses like brie, camembert, feta and ricotta can also be contaminated.

It is important to wash hands, chopping boards and utensils before preparing foods. Listeria is heat-sensitive, so make sure food is hot when you reheat it.

Toxoplasmosis

Toxoplasmosis is caused by *Toxoplasma gondii*, a type of parasite spread by domestic cats and kittens after they eat infected rodents or birds. The parasites are shed in the cat's poo and take one to five days to become infectious. Humans are infected by contact with contaminated kitty litter or soil.

I am a cat lover, but I would advise you not to get a new cat while pregnant. Old cats are safer. If you have a cat, keep it inside. Get someone else to change the kitty litter daily or wear gloves and wash your hands when doing this task.

To reduce the risk of toxoplasmosis you should wash vegetables prior to eating or preparing them and cook meat well.

Infection during pregnancy may not cause any obvious symptoms. But, your baby is still at risk of congenital toxoplasmosis. Even if there is no obvious disease at birth, your baby can develop a fever, rash, jaundice (yellow eyes and skin) and large liver and spleen.

Some babies have a very small head and seizures. If untreated, they can have long-term disability due to eye and brain damage and severe hearing difficulty. The most common late finding is damage to the eye resulting in vision loss called chorioretinitis.

Syphilis

Congenital syphilis is less frequent now due to routine antenatal screening which detects serological evidence of this sexually transmitted infection. You can contract syphilis if you have had sexual contact or intercourse with an infected partner without taking precautions such as using condoms. Some women don't know they have been infected with syphilis until it is detected with a positive blood test.

Syphilis is caused by the spirochete *Treponema pallidum*. It is treated with antibiotics, usually a form of penicillin, given by injection.

If your baby is infected with syphilis while still inside the uterus it can be stillborn or born prematurely (early). Babies born with congenital syphilis can be asymptomatic at birth but develop long-term complications. Education regarding the nature of STIs remains an important preventive public health issue for women of childbearing age.

Rubella (German measles)

Congenital rubella syndrome is fortunately rare in our country because of effective childhood immunisation programs. They include the combined MMR vaccine for measles, mumps and rubella. Although rubella is a mild disease in children, it has devastating effects on the developing foetus if contracted by a non-immune pregnant mother. Clinical consequences of this disease to the baby include brain damage, blindness, deafness and heart abnormalities.

Women who are not immunised should receive the MMR vaccine at least 28 days before becoming pregnant. This vaccine is a live attenuated vaccine, so cannot be given during pregnancy or to someone who has a problem with their immune system.

Our National Immunisation Program provides 'flu shots' for pregnant women during any stage of their pregnancy. It now funds and recommends the administration of the adult DTPa (diphtheria-tetanus–acellular pertussis) vaccine in the third trimester of pregnancy to protect mothers and babies from whooping cough, a potentially fatal neonatal infection.

Outbreaks of childhood illnesses such as pertussis (whooping cough) can place your newborn baby at risk. Unprotected babies who are too young to be immunised still die from this respiratory illness. Yet, some parents don't immunise their children.

We have had high levels of what is termed 'herd immunity', a form of collective community protection against specific diseases. This occurs when the majority of people immunise their children against potentially serious childhood infections. This has largely protected people who for medical reasons cannot be immunised and those who choose not to immunise or elect homeopathic immunisation. As the level of herd immunity drops, the risk of potential infection from rubella, measles and even polio increases.

Cytomegalovirus (CMV)

Cytomegalovirus (CMV) is the most common congenital viral infection, occurring in about 6 in 1,000 of live births. Most of these infections are asymptomatic at delivery with only about 10 per cent showing clinical evidence of disease. But, around 1 in 1,000 live births have permanent morbidity due to hearing loss, vision impairment, cerebral palsy, intellectual disability, seizures and even death.

Many women will have had CMV infection prior to pregnancy and have a lesser risk of passing the infection to their baby. The greatest risk is for mothers who get CMV in the first half of their pregnancy. CMV is not part of routine antenatal screening unless a pregnant mother develops an acute viral illness or has a foetal abnormality on ultrasound.

CMV is common in young children and therefore childcare workers planning a pregnancy should take extra caution by careful hand washing when changing nappies, helping children blow their noses or assisting with toileting duties. Women of childbearing age who have not had a CMV infection should not share food, drinks, utensils or toothbrushes with young children in their care.

Herpes simplex virus (HSV)

HSV infection is extremely common. There are two types. Type 1 causes recurrent cold sores. It can also be transferred to the genital area. Type 2 causes genital herpes and is considered a sexually transmitted infection. It can be asymptomatic – you don't know you are infected. Or, present with ulcers or abrasions in the genital tract or buttock area. If a woman has an active HSV lesion which is shedding virus and not recognised during labour, she can pass this infection to her baby at the time of delivery. Let your obstetrician or midwife know if you have had a genital HSV infection. If you have an active lesion or the start of one, as indicated by a localised tingling or burning sensation of your skin around the time of labour, inform your obstetric carer.

Sometimes women don't tell their partner about a previous genital HSV infection. If this applies to you, it is best to have already had this conversation with your obstetrician. They can guide you through this dilemma in a confidential manner.

Suppressive oral antiviral therapy such as acyclovir is prescribed from 36 weeks of gestation. This reduces the likelihood of HSV recurrence at the onset of labour. Caesarean delivery is protective and recommended if an active lesion is present at the time of anticipated delivery. If the possibility of having HSV is causing you undue anxiety and spoiling your pregnancy experience, discuss having an elective caesarean section. Stress is bad for pregnant mothers and just as bad for unborn babies. There are women who have a legitimate 'social' reason for electing a surgical birth. We should not be judgemental about their decision.

HSV congenital infection presents with minimal or non-specific symptoms such as poor feeding, temperature instability and early breathing problems. Serious sequelae include shock due to rapid drops in blood pressure and bleeding problems. A baby can have an apnoea, which means it stops breathing and turns blue or pale in colour and its heart rate will slow. Ongoing infection is either localised to the skin, eyes, mouth or central nervous system or widespread, involving multiple organs.

It is important to maintain perspective as your baby has only a small likelihood of having a serious infectious illness. You worry about all the things that can go wrong in a pregnancy. Remember that mostly things go right. HSV infection, for example, affects as few as five or less babies in every 100,000 deliveries in Australia. Higher figures apply for babies born in the US.

Varicella zoster (chicken pox)

Varicella infection is very contagious prior to the emergence of the typical chicken pox rash and until no new skin lesions erupt and all existing lesions have scabbed over. It has an incubation period of up to 21 days. If a non-immune mother comes into contact with chicken pox before 20 weeks of pregnancy or gets it from 7 days prior to or 28 days after delivery, the baby is at risk of developing a significant disease. The risk of mortality (death) is up to 30 per cent. If you have not had chicken pox but are exposed to this infection whilst pregnant, you must get medical advice. The administration of zoster immunoglobulin (ZIG) within 72 hours of exposure gives some protection to pregnant women with a history of chicken pox contact.

Newborn babies have an immature immune system and thin skin which makes them more vulnerable to infection. Until a baby receives its first immunisations at 8 weeks of age it is best to avoid exposing your baby to obvious infection. This can be difficult, particularly if you have other young children. Visitors who have the flu, chicken pox or a chronic repetitive cough that could be whooping cough should wait until they are well before visiting your baby.

HIV infection
This is a viral infection which attacks the immune system. In its most advanced stage it is known as AIDS. The virus is transmitted by infected blood and sexual secretions. In 1 to 2 per cent of cases, it is transferred from an infected mother to her unborn or newly delivered baby. Breastfeeding is discouraged in an infected mother.

HIV can be asymptomatic or present with fever, rash, headaches, muscle aches and pains, and enlarged lymph nodes. Blood tests can detect and monitor this virus. Treatment is with expensive antiretroviral medication. This is given to infants to try to prevent the transmission of HIV from their mother.

Zika virus

Infection in adults from this virus, known as a flavivirus, is asymptomatic or presents as fever, a slightly itchy rash, aching joints and conjunctivitis. 'Zika' is carried by mosquitoes and transmitted by their bite. It can also be transferred by sex, blood transfusion and organ transplant.

Women who contract Zika virus during pregnancy can pass the infection to their unborn child. It is controversial but accepted that this infection causes microcephaly (abnormally small heads), brain damage, foetal loss or stillbirth.

Group B streptococcus (GBS)

Group B streptococcus (GBS) is a major cause of infection in newborn babies, presenting early, within the first seven days, or late from one to three months. Babies present with fever, fast and laboured breathing, lethargy and pallor. They can rapidly progress to life-threatening infections of the blood or brain, such as meningitis. Severe GBS disease can cause the rapid demise of the baby and death within a few hours, even when antibiotics are given.

Severe streptococcal infection occurred more commonly in the past. It is seen less since screening and proactive treatment have been adopted. However, babies can still die from this bacterial infection. We can never be complacent about it. GBS screening between 35 and 37 weeks and preventive measures during pregnancy and labour have significantly reduced this potentially devastating bacterial infection.

Women who have previously screened positive for GBS from uterine or vaginal swabs or have delivered a baby affected by GBS are managed as high risk. They receive antibiotics, usually a form of penicillin, in early labour. Prophylactic treatment is not required for women who have an elective caesarean section, are not in labour and have not ruptured their membranes.

Around 15 to 25 per cent of women have asymptomatic carriage of GBS. If untreated, this would result in 1 in 200 neonates developing severe infection known as neonatal sepsis. The use of antibiotics such as penicillin or ampicillin for these women during labour has significantly reduced the incidence of early GBS disease in babies. This is a good thing!

Pneumococcal disease

Streptococcus pneumoniae bacteria or pneumococcus causes severe illness such as pneumonia, meningitis, and ear and blood infections. The very young, the elderly and those with their spleen removed are most at risk.

Treatment is with antibiotics and acute medical care. Pneumococcal vaccination is the best prevention for this serious disease. It is part of the National Immunisation Program Schedule.

ACKNOWLEDGEMENTS

To parent, teach, care and mentor a child is almost as difficult as writing a book. I could not have written *Parenting is Forever* without the unconditional love of my parents, Jan and Barry. I am grateful that my two daughters are proud of their mum, although somewhat incredulous that I know anything about being a good parent. My husband, Stephen Langford, threw down the gauntlet when he wrote his wonderful book, *The Leading Edge: Innovation, technology and people in Australia's Royal Flying Doctor Service.* He encouraged me to find the book hidden in my manuscript and to keep knocking on publishers' doors.

Thank you to Terri-ann White, publisher from UWAP, who opened the door, took a step out of her comfort zone and embraced a book about children. To the team at UWAP who sprinkle their magic on a manuscript and give it a voice and a presence, my gratitude and respect.

To name mentors, teachers and good friends risks the oversight of many compassionate people who have guided my career and life path. I will regret the omissions, but hope that those named will link with others who have made a difference to me and to my family.

I thank my school teachers; especially my Year 5 teacher at Kununurra Primary, my Year 4 teacher Anne McDonald, Albert Manning from Gunning Primary in NSW and Miss Eglite who taught me French at Ivanhoe Girls' Grammar School in Melbourne.

My medical and surgical mentors also wrote the textbooks I studied from: Professor Ken Hardy, Professor Norman Beischer, Professor Gab Kovacs, Professor Gordon Clunie and Professor Richard Lovell. As an intern at the Royal Melbourne Hospital I learned so much from two awesome doctors, Carlos Scheinkestel and Tom Kay.

I am grateful for the privilege of being a flying doctor in Kalgoorlie and working with Indigenous communities in the Western Desert. This was the first time I felt like a 'real doctor'. It was when I knew I had to be a paediatrician and care for children.

I am a paediatrician because of creative thinkers like 'Bush Bishop' Howell Witt and great clinicians: Grant Barham, Michael Pain, Rex Henderson, Trevor Parry, Peter Chauvel, Lou Landau, Geoff Byrne, Tim Jones, Paddy Pemberton, Noel French, Corrado Minutillo, David O'Donovan, Jacqui Scurlock, Kay Johnston, Paul Carman, Alan Duncan, Tony Keil, Peter Walsh, Jon Silberstein, Geoff Lam, Luigi D'Orsogna and Jim Ramsay. And, because Josephine (Jo) Sauvarin, dared me to do something different with my life.

My two loyal secretaries Bev and Carole and my amazing support person, Jan, have made it possible for me to continue my work as a paediatrician. My extended family, compassionate neighbours, friends, colleagues, and book club and tennis ladies make life a positive journey.

It is our adult responsibility to believe, prioritise and value childhood. To respect and be kind to children. When I was rostered to attend the delivery of sick newborn babies and had to crawl out of bed at 2 am, my husband would say, 'It's not the baby's fault'. That simple call to duty has kept me going for over 20 years. I am humbled to reflect that I may have made a difference.

I thank all those parents and families who have trusted me with their baby, child, adolescent or young adult.

ACKNOWLEDGEMENTS

The author gratefully acknowledges the permission granted to reproduce the copyright material in this book.

Guess How Much I Love You by Sam McBratney and illustrated by Anita Jeram published by Walker Books, 1994.

Oh the Places You'll Go by Dr Seuss published by Random House, 1990.

The Bug
Words and Music by Mark Knopfler
Copyright © 1990 Chariscourt Ltd.
International Copyright Secured All Rights Reserved
Reprinted by Permission of Hal Leonard LLC

The Cat in the Hat Comes Back by Dr Seuss published by Random House, 1958.

The Normal Child: Some Problems of the Early Years and Their Treatment by Ronald Illingworth published by Churchill Livingstone, 1991.

'This Be The Verse' by Philip Larkin from *The Complete Poems by Philip Larkin* published by Faber and Faber Ltd, 2014.

'Worstward Ho' by Samuel Beckett from *Nohow On* by Samuel Becket published by Grove Press, 2014.

Every effort has been made to trace the copyright holders and obtain permission to reproduce this material. Please do get in touch with any enquiries or any information relating to this material or the rights holder.

INDEX

Lightning Source UK Ltd.
Milton Keynes UK
UKHW040732100822
407113UK00004B/1183